A Prescription for Patience

— • —

A Message from the Publisher

In keeping with White Knight Publication's mandate
to bring great titles of social value to the reading public
across North America, we feel indeed fortunate as a dedicated
non-fiction publisher to have been closely involved
with this important publication that will originate
White Knight's latest genre,
"The White Knight Health Series"

A Prescription for Patience

A guide to improving our healthcare system!

by

Dr. Kevin J. Leonard, B.Comm, MBA, Ph.D., CMA

Associate Professor, Faculty of Medicine, University of Toronto
Research Scientist, Centre for Global eHealth Innovation,
University Health Network, Toronto, CANADA

The New White Knight Health Series

White Knight Publications
Toronto Canada

Published in 2005 by White Knight Publications,
a division of Bill Belfontaine Ltd.
Suite 103, One Benvenuto Place
Toronto Ontario Canada M4V 2L1
T. 416-925-6458 F. 416-925-4165
E-mail: whitekn@istar.ca
Web site: www.whiteknightpub.com

Ordering information

CANADA
Hushion House Publishing Inc.
c/o Georgetown Terminal Warehouses
34 Armstrong Avenue,
Georgetown ON, L7G 4R9
T: 1-866-485-5556 F: 1-866-485-6665

UNITED STATES
Hushion House Publishing Inc.
c/o Stackpole Distribution
7253 Grayson Road
Harrisburg PA, 17111 USA
T: 1-888-408-0301 F: 1-717-564-8307

National Library of Canada Cataloguing in Publication

Leonard, Kevin J., 1957–
        A prescription for patience : a guide to keeping our
        healthcare system healthy! / Kevin J. Leonard.

ISBN 0-9736705-1-7

1. Medical care—Canada. 2. Patient satisfaction—Canada.
I. Title.

RA395.C3L46 2005   362.1'0971   C2005-901507-1

Cover and text design: Karen Petherick, *Intuitive Design International Ltd.*
Typeset in: Janson
Editing: Penny Hozy
Cover photos: © Life Stock Photos

Printed and Bound in Canada

DEDICATION AND ACKNNOWLEDGEMENTS

Like all other literary ventures that I have been a part of, there are many people who are behind the scenes that offer tremendous support – support without which the project would have come to a screeching halt. This book is no exception.

I would like to dedicate this book to my mother who spent literally countless hours nursing me back to health, time and time again. At age fourteen, when no one believed that I was suffering from a mysterious illness, she was the sole source of comfort because I knew that she *knew* that I was ill. After many doctor visits and hours sitting in the waiting room, her resilience and dedication paid off in my finally obtaining the proper diagnosis and the correct treatment. I believe that her everlasting gift to me will always be her determination – no struggle is too hard. Perhaps the best part of all is that she says she did "just what *any* mother would do for her child." Thank you, for doing it!

I have had many teachers who spent many hours helping me improve my writing skills over the years and to them I say, I hope I have justified your faith in me. A few names deserve special attention – Luana Berard, George Khouri, Tony Parr, Martin Kusy, Mohsen Anvari, Jerry Tomberlin, Derek Diorio, Leslie O'Dell and Bruce Dow.

As well, as you will read throughout this book, I have been actively involved with many industries. I could not possibly have made the contributions in these many areas of my life without people helping and believing in me and in my crazy ideas. Once again, special recognition goes to – Doug Kinnear, George Osborne, Bill Osborne, Dale Doreen, Rawy Shediac, Latimer Asch, John Riley, David Bloom, Bruno Tenaglia, Roger Neilson, Ron Smith, Pat Quinn, Lorna Marsden, Gerald Keller, Tom Honey, Kevin Mercer, Peggy Leatt, George Pink, Stephen Sheather, Alex Jadad, Calvin Lei, Stephen Wolman, Peter Rossos and John Wright.

Finally, you fight the many battles that I have fought for one main reason – and in this area I am not unique – for your family. To all of my family (my mother, father, brother, sister and their families; and to Sandra, Noel and Randall), who carried me when I needed it most, thank you for your support. In the end, you were my greatest teachers!

CONTENTS

Dr. Kevin Leonard is uniquely positioned to prescribe change for our healthcare system. His personal challenge with illness, business expertise and academic background allow him to view healthcare delivery from a unique, multifaceted perspective.

His book is valuable reading for healthcare providers, administrators, politicians and all other individuals interested in healthcare access and delivery. Patients with chronic illness and their families could benefit from the perspective and personal anecdotes offered by Dr. Leonard.

The appropriate use of information technology can improve access and quality of care. Chronic illness accounts for the burden of healthcare costs and services in industrialized nations. An integrated electronic health record and remote care strategy could assist individuals challenged by chronic illness to achieve their personal and professional goals through improved treatment compliance, health promotion, reduction of clinical visits, and communication with and among care providers.

Progressive lack of hospital and community-based resources for services such as hemodialysis, postoperative care, post-transplant management and other complicated medical illnesses has created the need for increased patient involvement in disease management and prevention.

In Canada, national harmonization of services and health records is complicated by provincial jurisdiction over funding, legislation and licensing. Regionalized service coordination is frequently absent. Hospital and community-based care are often fragmented, resulting simultaneously in redundant provision and lack of service accessibility. The existing political and medical infrastructure has achieved limited success in addressing these challenges to date.

Consumers and providers of healthcare must drive change. Clinical necessity, technical capacity and cost-effectiveness will ultimately serve to overcome implementation issues related to licensing, reimbursement and medico-legal considerations. Well-informed patient advocates and their care providers must drive this initiative from a grass roots level.

I am honoured to share this vision with Dr. Leonard. We have arrived at this common point from opposite ends of the healthcare spectrum. As our population progressively ages, many more of us will acquire chronic illnesses requiring management in a financially challenged system. Fortunately, the appropriate application of information technology may help us in our personal and societal goals to live well and independently.

Peter G. Rossos, M.D., F.R.C.P.(C)
Associate Professor of Medicine, University of Toronto
Program Director, University of Toronto Division of Gastroenterology
Director of Medical Informatics, University Health Network

Over the last thirty years or so, I have had the opportunity to spend a significant amount of time as a patient in hospitals and at home receiving home care treatment. Although the negatives associated with a lifelong chronic condition are obvious, my illness has provided me with the opportunity to grow personally beyond my years and to learn how to value each and every day. I was once told that I am very difficult to work with because I want to do everything I can every day – I cannot wait until tomorrow. In other words, I treat every day like it's my last. I think that may have been the greatest compliment I have ever received.

More importantly, however, my illness has forced me to spend time with health providers thereby allowing me to see first-hand what it's like to be a patient. Communication inefficiencies are our most glaring problem. Having to go into a hospital on a continuing basis is extremely frustrating and debilitating enough; having to provide all of our demographic details, as well as our complete medical history, each and every time we see a new provider, is incredibly agonizing. Has it ever occurred to the medical profession that sometimes the patient just does not *want* to have to relive all of the problems again by relaying them to a new group of providers each time?

Further, it should be recognized that every time patients relay their history, the likelihood of it being incomplete, inconsistent or incorrect goes up dramatically.

In the healthcare industry, the main premise of new technologies for information systems is that the increased utilization of computers would benefit the healthcare system in many ways. First, it would streamline costs by reducing redundancy of tests and prescriptions. Second, it could increase efficiencies of delivery of service within hospitals by providing faster and more accurate data and information on patients. Third, incorporating a collaborative attitude toward information management in community care agencies could affect increased efficacy and improve patient and staff satisfaction throughout the entire healthcare system.

It is my belief that the main benefit from the implementation of computer systems in healthcare, in addition to improved efficiency, is the potential for improvement in effectiveness. The theory goes something like this: Doctors get data and information on their patients faster because all of their files of treatments and diagnoses are computerized and can be retrieved electronically and almost instantly. This then allows for better health management because treatment decisions, for example, are based on complete information about the patient.

Better health management should lead to a healthier patient on an individual basis as well as creating improved health outcomes (i.e., effectiveness) across the system as a whole. Furthermore, effective treatments can lead to a reduction in the number of services required, thereby reducing costs. In addition, computers can play a large role by providing management information on where there are inefficiencies in service delivery throughout healthcare today. Although there has been very little research to date tying in the adoption of new technology to improved healthcare outcomes, this is a research hypothesis that I truly believe in. Personally, I know of many times that I suffered needlessly because my doctors could not get the information that *I desperately needed*. This must become the ultimate goal of new technology in healthcare – improved health outcomes.

To this end, public concern for confidentiality and security of health information must be heard and addressed. *We must have a concerted public input into the current status of healthcare!* This will allow citizens to be given a forum to address general overall health delivery concerns such as gaps in service. We have to ensure that patients are invited to the discussion in order to join the healthcare organizations, providers and government in setting policy and putting plans into action. Without understanding which services are providing the most value to its customers (i.e., the patients), effective change management will be impossible to achieve.

If (or, hopefully, when) we attain this goal of improved information systems, then, and only then, will we have satisfied a necessary condition for a healthcare system that allows the patients to move seamlessly between the various healthcare providers without the need to spend valuable time providing demographic and historical healthcare data at each stop. This book describes the steps that need to be taken to ensure that information systems are designed, developed and implemented in the most effective manner possible. Moreover, this book uses my experience both in the Canadian and American healthcare systems as the context for this discussion; however, the issues and development that must take place are relevant to all settings for healthcare delivery globally today. In the chapters that follow, this generalizability will be explored in order to high-light the importance of the solutions that we can and must all create together.

I truly hope that you will find this book educational, enter-taining and inspiring. If I must leave you with only one thought, then it is this: If you believe in something, truly believe it, then never let go and never give in – whether it is a creative idea or just knowing that your child is sick. You may be proven wrong eventually but that is the only way you learn, by winning, or losing, on your own terms! Look at it this way, being proven wrong is a much better outcome than wondering forever what might have been.

CHAPTER ONE

The role of patients in our healthcare system

"You must be the change you wish to see in the world"
– Mahatma Gandhi

January 18, 1988 • *Ottawa, Ontario*

As I sat in the car and turned on the ignition, I knew I had only a couple of minutes before I passed out and stop breathing altogether. My breaths became shorter and none of my asthma medication was having any effect. I did not know the cause of this attack – however, I did know that I needed help immediately. I drove as fast as possible to the closest emergency room. I went through three stop signs and two red lights. A car was backing out of its driveway – which forced me to drive onto someone's lawn to avoid waiting; any additional minute could cost me my life. As I approached the hospital, I debated how to contact the emergency staff. Do I park the car and walk casually to the door – no time! Do I drive through the emergency room door, certain to get their attention –

too dramatic! I decided to lean on the horn.

This proved very effective. A wheelchair was brought out of the emergency department (ED) door just as I pulled in – perhaps only ten seconds after I initially hit the car horn. I managed to tell a doctor that I had allergies and asthma and he pieced together the rest. I passed out almost immediately thereafter. On my passage to mental oblivion, I felt the medical staff pulling off my clothes like there was no tomorrow.

When I awoke, almost 90 minutes later, the medical staff, after first convincing themselves that I was fine, started to reprimand me. First of all, I should be carrying a medical alert bracelet – if I had not been able to remain conscious to advise them of my condition, there was no limit to the possible causes for my condition and the cause for me to black out, hence treatment options would be risky. Second, I should be carrying an epinephrine kit (with a loaded syringe) that could be injected at the onset of the reaction. This would then have avoided the whole incident altogether. I was then briefed on the costs to the healthcare system when someone acts irresponsibly.

The physician kept me in hospital overnight and I was not allowed to leave in the morning until I had filled out the forms for a medical alert tag. I resented being talked to as if I were a child, incapable of managing my own affairs; however, he was absolutely correct – I took their help for granted – and that was to be a great lesson for me about the value of our health delivery system. You see, I was given a glimpse of the big picture, something that I had not yet been fortunate enough to see. When the doctors and nurses worked on me to "bring me back" and save my life, I was taking their time (skills and expertise) away from some other patient(s) who also needed that level of care. This resulted in reduced quality of treatment for them and/or me, and certainly in higher overall healthcare system costs. My irresponsible behaviour (due to my ignorance, but irresponsible nonetheless) put other factors and other people at risk! I vowed that day that I would repay the healthcare system for my irresponsibility – no matter how long or how much it took.

— • —

THE GLOBAL PATIENT

In most countries, the patients comprise both ends of the spectrum in the healthcare system; they are the payer of the system (either on their own, through their insurance premiums or government taxes) and are representative of the final customer (or patient). For example, in Canada taxpayer dollars almost entirely fund healthcare services. This is unique when compared to other industries. In most, there are companies and organizations that invest in a product or service delivery and then the consuming public decides whether or not to spend their money within that industry. In healthcare, the investment comes directly from the public, which also comprises the consumer base. As a result, one would expect that patients, as a group, would be involved in both the use and the *management* of the healthcare system. However, this is not the case; patients have not been involved in either the management of the system or of their own health.

Is it because the system runs itself so well that we don't need to get involved? In short, this is highly unlikely as the system is operating very poorly! If we were getting the same level of "respect" or "service" from any other industry or institution, we would all gather together, organize and form a boycott to demand improvement. At the very least, we would not think twice about voicing our individual points of view, seeking attention from the industry and investigating alternatives.

As an example, if a bank manager kept changing appointment times and advising you that he did not have any data about your mortgage renewal (principal outstanding, interest rate, term and payment amount), you would approach that bank manager and demand changes. Or, you would go to another institution that would respect your business more. However, in healthcare, these very things are occurring all the time and we choose, individually and collectively, to say nothing. Access to our own comprehensive health record is non-existent. It's next to impossible to have a complete listing of all of our drugs, diagnosis and outcomes on a historical basis – on paper, online or otherwise. Imagine your bank, trust company or credit union having no idea what your balance was and how much it had changed since last year, last month or last week – would you not want to see the president?

Patients have to get more involved in the management of their own care – and especially now. At present, our healthcare investment or overall system survival is definitely in jeopardy. With nurses and other caregivers losing jobs through budget cuts and services moved to other, often distant and inconvenient locations, our health risk has increased dramatically. Yet, to date, we have said nothing. With movement to electronic patient records in the future, one would think that patients would be leading the debate about this change and the impact on confidentiality versus the risk of no information at all. Yet we choose not to participate in the process of reform. This change and progress must occur and the system must evolve. I also believe, however, that patients *must* be involved in this process in order to make sure that their voices can be heard and issues protected.

The need for the patient perspective is also evident at the system level across all types of healthcare structures (e.g., insurance based in the US or the socialized medicine in Canada). Due to a significant "power differential" that exists between clinicians and patients all around the world, most patients are too intimidated to exercise their collective input. Whether the payer is the province (as in Canada), a large health management organization (HMO as in the US), insurance companies or the patients themselves, the patient-doctor relationship plays itself out the same, with patients being extremely reluctant to question the system. The key message here is that the healthcare system does require questioning. It can and must be improved if it is to survive.

THE CANADIAN EXAMPLE

In Canada, for example, socialized medicine is considered to be one of the most sacred rights – a part of the national fabric. The vast majority of Canadians believe in this concept that was started by the Tommy Douglas New Democratic Party (NDP) in Saskatchewan in the late 1950s. A healthcare system that prescribes universal access, regardless of social status, that is paid for totally from public funds. Canadians believe in the five basic tenets of the Canada Health Act (last revised in 1984): universality, accessibility, comprehensiveness, portability, and accountability. However, even this system that is considered the envy of many other countries requires change; it needs an update; it demands improvement. At the moment, this is a system that is in jeopardy of collapsing due to both economic and clinical strain. Some of this stress must be relieved from the system and this can only be accomplished by patients sharing some of the management burden.

Canada is facing the possibility of a two-tiered system; the possibility of the rich being able to opt out of a public system and pay for services that they and only they can afford and fund. Once this becomes achieved, and thereby acceptable, growth in a two-tiered system will only be a matter of degree as opposed to a matter of national philosophy and cultural principles. In some ways, Canadians have already moved to a two- (some might even say multi-) tiered system that does not treat people equally. One good example is people's social class and their informal network of connections allowing them to get to see doctors faster than others might – this is happening *today* – is this the system Canadians want?

The concept of a two-tiered system as discussed here should not be confused with the private versus public debate that is also taking place in boardrooms and living rooms around the country. There is nothing contrary to the Canada Health Act about private for-profit organizations treating patients as long as it is entirely funded by the public purse. If every patient gets treated and no personal funds exchanged, then all that is happening is that organizations with experience running a process efficiently are now getting the chance to help out our healthcare system. Not only should this not be feared, it should be applauded – we need all the help we can get. The two-tiered system, on the other hand, is one where people are required to pay for services that are offered else-where for free.

One might ask, what's wrong with a two-tiered system? If the rich want to opt out of one system and go to another that they pay for, then why should I care as long as my system is left alone? And therein lies the problem – the publicly funded system will not be left alone because there are limited resources, with these limited resources being primarily human in nature. In other words, the best doctors, surgeons, nurses and therapists will be attracted to the privately funded system where there will be better facilities, better working conditions and, presumably, better wages. The publicly funded system will quickly become a second-class system. The objective must be to improve the current universal healthcare system to the point where we *all* have access to better facilities and better conditions – and it must be done now!

What changes are needed? How do we, as patients, go from where we are today to this improved healthcare system that is needed? How do we do that without destroying the principles that we all hold so dear?

The final answers to these questions must be *determined* by all of the health stakeholders together, mainly because the "best" answers are not straightforward. It's not obvious to the healthcare industry (or anyone, for that matter) what the optimal system should look like, let alone how to get there. The main drawbacks are both a lack of vision and a lack of information. Doctors, hospitals and even governments cannot determine what works well and what does not work well in healthcare systems today. They cannot tell us which hospitals perform which specific tasks better than other hospitals. They can give us some information about length of stay, for example, but cannot calculate costs and outcomes at the patient level or related to specific stays. Therefore, as an example, one cannot translate length of stay to quality of care.

Yet, many healthcare organizations are desperately trying to shorten length of stay across a wide array of disease categories. However, there is no guarantee that shortened lengths of stay will reduce costs. Obviously, costs are reduced if patients go home faster but, if they go home too early, there may be significant costs incurred when/if the patient comes back and gets re-admitted. Secondly, home care costs may go up more than hospital costs go down, primarily due to the fact that when a patient goes home early, the cost cutting is on the most inexpensive in-hospital days, ones at end of stay when the patient requires less services than the average patient.

Therefore, overall health system costs may, in fact, go up, and doubly so if the beds are then re-populated with sicker patients. Thirdly, home care is often not covered under the health insurance plans, so much of the actual home care costs go unrecognized and unmeasured ... causing a large burden on families and other informal health support networks, thereby adding a further cost to the overall management of health. By how much? Unfortunately, governments and ministries of health cannot calculate this number any more than anyone else because of the lack of information around the comprehensiveness of these costs.

Other areas of healthcare provide similar levels of inadequate information. Hospital administrators are uncertain how to evaluate their performances across a wide level of indices for many reasons. First, there is no standardization of how these indices should be calculated or interpreted. Second, there is no forum for comparison, thus no benchmark to evaluate against. Finally, information is so difficult to get at that whatever information is calculated gets delivered so long "after the fact," it's no longer useful. Without access to information, effective evaluation is impossible!

THE PATIENT'S PERSPECTIVE

To date, all of the other stakeholders in healthcare have been involved in the management of the system. The doctors and nurses have well-coordinated organizations that effectively and independently represent their interests. The provincial, state and national hospital associations represent the hospitals; and the government involvement is legendary. However, no one ever thinks to involve the public. It is ironic since this sector is the biggest player in our healthcare system. To repeat, not only are we the finished product (in a manner of speaking), but we are the full payers of the system as well. You'd think that someone would have invited the public to the meetings before now!

To some degree, many will argue, the public has been involved through government, lobby groups or representation on hospital boards or community service groups and

committees. But, for the most part, these "so-called represen-
tations" reflect a small interest group or act with total
independence. There is no real health group that has managed
to organize and represent the will of the general public – the
sick *and* the healthy. This is desperately needed. If not
accomplished soon, then many of the decisions will be made
without patient involvement.

Why have we not tried to organize before now? To this
end, a meeting was called a couple of years ago in Kitchener–
Waterloo, Ontario, in order to raise public awareness and to
"get the patient contribution organized." This meeting was
advertised through the large regional newspaper and through
the local District Health Council. Unfortunately, only six
people from the general public showed up. Apparently, very
little word had spread. I believe that the public is more interested than they have exhibited so far.

Why is it that we only get involved when what we have
today is threatened? It appears to be some kind of perverse
human behaviour to fight only for something when someone
is taking it away – as opposed to when they are just *threatening*
to take it away. It would appear to me that the earlier the
involvement the better. If you are involved in the discussions
from the very beginning, then you can have a greater effect on
the design of the solution. Additionally, when stakeholder
groups are involved there is a greater feeling of ownership (or
buy-in) that helps increase the likelihood of success.

Alternatively, we do not seem to react with the same verve
when we are discussing the change to, or the removal of,
services that we are not using or do not yet have access to.
Again, it seems that we only fight for what we have right now
and only when it is being removed or changed – at the time of

the change – not beforehand. Why else do we have so many strikes and labour strife that only get settled during last-minute negotiations?

A good example of this is in sports. The field of sports is very attractive for analysis because all components in life are involved – except often the process is quickened tremendously, resulting in an explosion of emotions. We have wins and losses, good bosses and bad ones, close friends and those teammates that let us down, strong supporters and those that leave us when things are going poorly. There is nothing that occurs in life that cannot be experienced in sports as well. Why do players not play with the same tenacity every game – why do they only play the best when they have to – when they are on the verge of losing something? We see the same phenomenon in all sports. The best games are always in the playoffs – and usually when one team (or both) is on the verge of elimination. How do we as coaches or as administrators get our players or employees excited about every day? How do we get the public interested in fighting for something *before* we lose it (perhaps) for good?

This activity or inactivity, on behalf of the general public, has led us to the point where we are now – and even now, when so much of healthcare that we hold so dear is about to change, even now, we are not *active* in the fight for healthcare survival. What will it take to get the public involved? Oh yes, we hear of a fight to save a hospital here or a clinic there, but once again, this is only at the time that the change is announced. Where are the people that should be active in the decision-making process? The input from the public is needed *now* before long-term decisions are made.

Is it that people are afraid to stand up and say what's right or wrong? Maybe we're all just too busy with our lives and are satisfied with others taking the lead and, if things don't go well, we're only too happy to criticize afterward.

Until now, as a society we have been extremely accepting. Whoever we happen to draw in the emergency room (ER) lottery is who we accept to handle our health problems. Is this the best procedure to follow?

Consider the following: We are visiting a friend's house and we suffer an allergic reaction to something we eat. We are rushed to the hospital – often the closest one. Who treats us? Whoever is "on call." We have very little choice.

Take a second example: We've had a nagging problem for some time, and then finally go to the emergency room at the hospital when the pain gets too severe – instead of seeing our General Practitioner (GP). In this case, it seems that we're managing our health only because we had to – we're not being proactive. Whatever doctor comes to treat us in the clinic or ER is the one that we accept. Then we scream when the procedure goes wrong. Did we see the person who was not the most qualified to help us or, perhaps, at the outset of the problem, should we have been treated by a different health professional?

In effect, we have managed the healthcare system in the same way that we manage our personal health ... we leave the most important decision making to others! When something comes up we allow it to be addressed by whomever and whatever is around. Regarding the system, if we become short of capital, we merge two hospitals that are close together (i.e., regionalization) or combine two hospitals that do the same thing (i.e., consolidation). Is this the right approach? Should we not be more strategic rather than reactionary? Should we not do our homework – analyze the data and information? Where is the information that we need to make these decisions?

So, if it's this obvious, why are patients not organizing together? In this book, I will illustrate the many reasons why we have put this public input off for so long. The bottom line is that we need to find the solution, to find the truth … as well as an answer to these questions: What is the best system for all patients; what does the "patient/public" want from our healthcare system; what are they willing to pay for? And these truths cannot be found by scurrying away from the debate or by performing another government-funded study. It must happen! All of us – everyone – must become more interested and involved in our healthcare system. This may mean anything from becoming more aware of the problems all the way up to actively campaigning for change.

We must begin to move forward and through this development, step by step. Many of the issues that need to be addressed can be addressed and overcome one at a time. But this will take time … which is why I have titled this book *A Prescription for Patience*. The key element is that we begin a journey today; a journey that may take ten years to complete. However, if we do not start today – since this necessary task will not go away – and we start only in five years time, then we will *still* be ten years away from creating the kind of health system we all want. We must begin now.

You may ask: What kind of system do we want? The answers are not straightforward – which is why we must solve this problem together. The change will happen with or without us – however, it is *much* more likely to be the system we want if we are involved.

How do we move forward? How can we get our voices heard? How do we make this debate happen? This book will show us how!

"The one person that will always have the greatest concern about their health and that of their family is the consumer. It's time to put the information necessary for the consumer to more effectively manage their healthcare in the hands of the consumer"

Brian Baum
CEO of Health Record Network Foundation,
Duke University School of Medicine.

CHAPTER TWO

Canada as a prototype for change

In many ways, Canada is a unique country. It is affluent as a nation, with technology sophistication rivaling that of the G8 nations. Yet, with only 32 million people in the second largest country in the world, in terms of landmass, there is a great opportunity to test out new solutions, new technology and communication methodologies. As such, its uniqueness provides an opportune platform to examine and learn from as Canada grows over time.

As I stated in the previous chapter, the patient stakeholder group must become more active in the healthcare industry. This activity will come in the form of consumerism, much like consumerism has changed the landscape of many industries over the last few decades. This impact has been made possible through evolving computerization and the growth and spread of new technology. Once consumers have a way "into an industry," then the power of the consumer cannot be ignored and must be addressed. I believe that it is this consumerism that is lacking in healthcare and this is a primary reason for the lack of information technology growth in healthcare. In this book, I will present Canada as an example of the effect that consumerism can have. Although the examples are

Canadian, the problem is global and issues relevant to all countries around the world.

I present the effect that consumers can have by discussing in some detail three very different industries; these industries are great examples because of their importance to Canadians. The three industries are: the banking industry, the educational system (at a university level), and professional hockey. I have been very fortunate to have worked in each of these industries and have attempted to be a change agent within each with varying degrees of success. As a result, I relate my experience and the effect that both changing technology and rising consumerism have had on these industries. The overall objective is, through the art of storytelling, to illustrate how each of these industries has dealt with adopting new information technology. Hopefully, these illustrations will provide valuable insight for healthcare.

To begin, I would like to explain how it is that I know so much about each of these industries. I was born and raised in Canada, studied at university level in Canada (undergraduate and post-graduate), have been a full-time lecturer at three Canadian Universities (received tenure in both a school of business and economics, and a faculty of medicine), worked with a Canadian National Hockey League (NHL) team, worked for both the central bank and a chartered bank in Canada and have run a consulting company in the financial services sector in this country. In addition, I have been employed by a consulting company in the United States of America and was a consultant for a US-based NHL team. Furthermore, I have lived in Montreal, Ottawa, Vancouver, Cambridge (Ontario), Kitchener–Waterloo, Toronto and in Marin County (just north of San Francisco). Therefore, I feel that I am qualified to talk about these four industries as well as to evaluate Canada's position with respect to other countries within each industry.

The banking industry in Canada is extremely efficient and is the envy of most countries around the world. The principal banks (the Schedule A banks) are all national banks and allow for very efficient transfer of funds and management of financial securities. Canada eliminated the concept of float long before many other countries by effectively exchanging money through the Bank of Canada each evening. Therefore, one can cash or deposit a cheque at one bank on Tuesday, drawn from a different bank's account, and by Wednesday, those funds are fully cleared through both banks.

The pride in Canada's banking system is exceeded by only three things: one of these is our love for hockey. Almost every Canadian boy (and more and more, Canadian girl) grows up and thinks of hoisting the Stanley Cup or of seeing his/her name on this prized trophy. Springtime is the time when Canadians hunker down in front of their televisions to watch the battle of the playoffs. Not only do they watch them, they're also very active in their interest – often exhibiting passion for the hometown teams at a level that rivals (if not exceeds) the level attached to most personal relationships.

Another valued treasure in Canada is the post-secondary education system. Canada has set its social policy such that every child in Canada that earns acceptance to a Canadian university can attend that university independent of his or her financial status. Their tuition fees are some of the lowest in the world and the quality of education is truly second to none. The federal government supports student tuition through the Canada Student Loan programs, which continually are improved every few years. The bottom line is that should one's grades be good enough, one can realistically choose to go to any university in the country. This is quite remarkable!

But perhaps its most valued social institution is Canada's healthcare system. It possesses many great characteristics – however, it's not perfect. The system has many flaws and as the baby boomers age and begin to stress the healthcare system in record numbers, these flaws could become cracks, ultimately with the potential to destroy the entire health delivery system. Unlike the other industries, healthcare does indeed affect all of us. We have all used the system and will all need to use the system in the future – in one way or another.

THE USE OF THE THREE INDUSTRIES

The best way to move people is through education. As an academic at Canada's largest university, I have dedicated my life to education because I truly believe that real change is only accomplished through education. In this book, I illustrate how technology (and the way we live our lives due to changing technology) has developed and affected the three example industries. I will inform and educate through my examples and interactions with these three industries (and hopefully entertain). I hope that these examples will help demonstrate how the same change can and will happen in healthcare and how important it is that we are all involved as this progresses.

It must be emphasized that this book is comprised solely of my theories and opinions based on my training and experience. I take great care to outline that experience so that one can better appreciate the commentary that is made herein. My recommendations are not solely my own, however, as they incorporate the input and writings of many others. What I present here is one synthesis, a synthesis that is greatly needed as technology adoption in practice and in research that is expanding at a pace that most of us just cannot comprehend.

I chose the education and banking industries because some of the conditions are very similar to healthcare. They both have serious issues related to security and confidentiality and they are both heavily information-based industries. They require the ability to network and the capacity to access information from multiple sites and in real time. Banking, in particular, being an industry that is run by for-profit corporations, has made much more progress than healthcare in effectively employing information technology. We can learn many lessons from their development – both positive and negative. Education, on the other hand, also publicly funded like healthcare, can illustrate an industry on the move driven by its consumers – the students.

I selected hockey as the example of a heavy consumer-based industry – which could also be represented by the entertainment sector, retail or any number of industries. It is perceived that the consumer has very little input into the development of this sector – being recipients rather than participants of the change or product that is being directed at them. The only real input they have is whether or not they accept or buy the product. However, this is a very powerful role and can have significant impact.

For each industry, I will describe the history through my interactions with this change and the role I have played around training, support and education. This will give an up-close look at how the industry has changed and will provide a common background for later discussions. We all have a tendency to look just at the current situation but my objective here is to show the history of chaos and resistance that stifled the change before the desire and need for improvement took over.

Secondly, I describe where we are today with respect to consumer expectations and how we can use this framework to our advantage – principally to evaluate the system and to use it to the best of our abilities or for the greatest possible gain. All of these industries are still evolving and it is very important to see the common positives and negatives – and, most importantly, to see and understand why. Further, since these industries are at different positions on the life cycle of change, analysis here will be most noteworthy.

The final component deals with performance measurement and how we must continue to grow and push these systems toward continuous improvement. We should not be happy with the status quo, no matter what that is. Everything can be improved, and we should learn how to get the improvement process started and keep it on track.

In summary, my personal mantra is "always keep demanding more!" – I told you I was tough to work with. Part of the problem in healthcare is that we have been very accepting of the status quo and not challenging the industry to do more.

There is an old story where a grandmother and grandson are walking down the beach talking about this and that. Out of nowhere, a giant wave rises up, hits the beach and grabs the grandson and pulls him into the ocean. The grandmother is stunned for a second, then – realizing what has happened – falls to her knees and starts screaming skyward. "Lord, Lord, just give me my grandson back; I'll do anything, please, please just bring him back alive." Once again, out of nowhere, a second wave rises up and spits the grandson back onto the beach. The grandmother gets to her feet, rushes over to her grandson and hugs him with all her might. She then looks skyward again and says: "Hey, he was wearing a hat!"

Always keep demanding more!

"The patient as expert and partner in care is an idea whose time has come and has the potential to create a new generation of patients who are empowered to take action to improve their health in an unprecedented way."

Liam Donaldson,
Chief Medical Officer, Department of Health,
London, England.

CHAPTER THREE

The critical success factors for adopting new technology

In this chapter, I present six critical success factors (of which, resistance to change is the first one) that must be addressed when adopting new technology. These factors can only be overcome through *work*; hence I present a technology adoption curve that outlines the workload or effort required to increase the likelihood of a successful adoption.

NEW TECHNOLOGY ADOPTION

Regardless of the industry, when change through the adoption of new technology takes place, the amount of work required to operate the existing system actually *increases*. This is always true and will last for a period of time. This may seem to be contrary to popular belief, which states that there should be efficiency (and even effectiveness) gains from new technology. Yes, this is true; once the new system has been implemented and working effectively, then efficiencies will increase – thereby reducing overall workload. However, during the *transition* or *adoption* of a new information system, the work increases and this increased work will last for a period of time. How much the work increases and the length of time depends on six critical success factors (CSFs), which are:

1. amount of resistance to change (i.e., presence of industry experience using the technology)
2. amount of training both before and during the transition (or implementation)
3. amount of buy-in (or contribution during design) from the different stakeholder groups
4. level of consumer (or end-user) influence during early stages of adoption
5. level of effective reporting on the status of the outcome measures during and post-implementation (i.e., communication on the technology adoption progress)
6. level of effectiveness in dealing with good or bad fortune (i.e., luck or the "breaks").

In some detail, if the industry in question and its personnel have had experience in using Information Technology (IT), then navigating its way through change management (and another similar adoption) or the job of providing "reasons for change" is made much easier. This is because the benefits are now known in advance and the industry has found ways either to address the resistance to change concerns or has learned how to deal with the obstacles.

Training is critical as new employees and even other more experienced personnel need support throughout the development and implementation life cycle. This training then provides stakeholders with the awareness, skills and confidence required to address concerns, overcome obstacles and ensure success.

The amount of stakeholder buy-in is normally attributed to the interaction between the system developers and the end users. The more the users are involved in the design and development of new information technology, the more they will perceive this new technology as "our own" system rather than one that was imposed on them from elsewhere.

The fourth CSF pertains to a stakeholder group that is very often overlooked – the end consumer. However, it is the consumer that has the most influence over whether a product or service is successful or not. Being able to engage consumers early in the adoption process is critical for new technology so that their perspectives and concerns are considered.

"Nothing succeeds like success!" These words were never more relevant than today in relation to IT adoption. The more progress we make the faster will be the next adoption. This critical factor promotes the idea that during adoption, stakeholders must be notified of the progress, which should be in the form of performance or outcome measures. This must happen as soon as possible after the intervention (or the implementation in this case) in order to sustain the momentum, the goodwill and the confidence.

Every person, every initiative has things that happen that were not planned and were outside the "scope of certain outcomes." Although these are not expected to happen, they still do occur; sometimes these things are positive and other times negative. The success of any project does not depend on whether the positives outweigh the negatives, but rather on how well the project leadership deals with these "breaks" in the first place.

We can examine the healthcare industry with respect to each of these six CSFs. There has been very little successful adoption of information technology throughout healthcare. As a result, the resistance to change factor has played a huge role. Further, there is a shortage of both experience and qualified trainers (leading to infrequent training) around the use of IT. During the historical episodic IT adoption, one of the main contributing factors to its poor success rate has been a lack of clinician stakeholder involvement. In addition, patients have very seldom been asked what information would be valuable to them. Next, there has been little, at least until just recently, accomplished in establishing performance metrics to evaluate the healthcare system in general. Therefore, relating an improvement in health outcomes (if there is one) back to IT investment has been extremely difficult. Keeping stakeholders apprised of this progress during and after implementation by reporting on these new metrics is still only a theoretical construct in today's healthcare environment. Finally, with more successful implementation of technology, the industry can only improve on dealing with both good and bad fortune as the sophistication of users increases.

Let us now examine the CSFs in the context of the amount of time and workload that is needed to be successful with IT adoption. Figure 1 represents this process graphically.

When technology is first introduced there is a certain amount of work still being expended to operate the current system – this is represented on the graph at Time 0, and should be considered as a "baseline workload level." At Time 1, a period of time has now gone by and the workload has increased to some degree. It is at this point that resistance to change starts to be articulated from the most ardent advocates of the why-fix-what-ain't-broke school of doing things. At Time 2, the workload is now increasing at an increasing rate and even the initial supporters of change are starting to have their

Figure 1

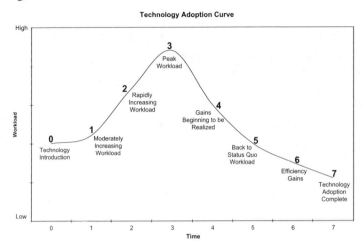

doubts; by the way, the system developers have begun to move loved ones out of town. At Time 3, information and computer system developers are among the most hated in society – second only to the people who draw up the instructions to those impossible-to-put-together toys; resistance to change groupies are now coming out of the woodwork … or wherever it is that they come out from. The *worst* words that a system engineer can hear are: "Do you know what 'waste of time' means?" It must be noted that if a system implementation is to fail it usually happens somewhere between Times 2 and 3 (although there are always exceptions).

At Time 4, the good guys start to win some public sentiment and there is the odd (usually very odd, in so many ways) comment that maybe things are not unsalvageable! By the time we reach Time 5 (if we reach Time 5), the systems engineers have now had their families return home, it's okay once again to say the individual names in public and overall morale has improved. As well, the total amount of workload using the new system is approximately about what it was under the old system

– we are once again at the "baseline workload level." The jobs and tasks have changed (often dramatically) but the total amount of work at least appears to be the same. Time 6 (and even more so at Time 7, if achieved) sees benefits improving at an increasing rate – often garnering wins in areas that were not even predicted when the system was first implemented. This is most often due to escalating effects and synergies. Here, people begin to realize the benefits and then create more opportunities, feeding off the first level benefits – creating new and continued avenues for growth and for working more cooperatively. The *best* words that any system developer can hear are: "Can you get the system to do this?" That is the precise moment you know that the audience of stakeholders has bought in to the vision!

Unfortunately, it is very difficult, in the abstract, to identify where an organization (or an industry, for that matter) is on this technology adoption curve or how long it will take to get to Time 4. Most of the people who resist change do not come up to the systems designers and say: "Your system is probably good and will help us in the long run, but I am very insecure, so could you please make all of this go away before I have a nervous breakdown!" If they did, then it would be easier to deal with them. What normally happens is that they preach about how bad things will be before the new system has ever been implemented. Then once implementation begins and the workload increases (which we know it must), they point to this as evidence that the system cannot work; often they say: "There was nothing really wrong with the old way" or employ any one of a series of endless asinine accusations. I refer to this as *aggressive ignorance*; there will always be people who resist change simply because it is change! In order to effectively challenge this we must realize that it is the change itself that they are aggressively fighting in order to remain ignorant.

If these resistors have any power whatsoever then the system will be shut down before it ever reaches Time 4. The only way to combat this attack from resistors is to find early adopters. These are people who like technology, embrace change and are not afraid of making mistakes. Every successful adoption of new technology has had supporters that ensured that the system had enough time to make it to Time 4 so that the positives could gain momentum and convert the resistors or, at the very least, remove their influence. These early adopters are often very creative in providing reasons for the change.

One fact relating to overcoming the resistance to change is that any type of technology change must be seen as being in one of two categories: either it is completely new technology whereby the benefits are obvious or can be easily and straight-forwardly articulated; or it is meant to replace existing technology and then it must (i) lower costs and/or (ii) improve the outcomes enough (either operationally or incrementally through the change) to justify the increased costs. A good example of the first is tele-medicine, which allows patients and clinicians to connect over long distances and has been very successful. The operational model is exactly the same as the traditional healthcare delivery model with the only difference being that patients can be evaluated and treated remotely. The technology adoption allows for this remote connectivity, which did not exist previously.

Most of the time, however, information technology is extremely difficult to justify because it is not of the first type above. Therefore, the new technology must either lower costs in the short-term – which we know it does not (see Figure 1)

– or it must improve outcomes – which we, as stated above, have a long history of not measuring or, at least, not with any consistency. Hence the dilemma: if we cannot demonstrate that new information technology has value, then to ensure successful adoption, we must become preachers of a new philosophy borrowed from W.P. Kinsella (*Shoeless Joe*, Mariner Books, 1982) – if you build it, they will come. Regrettably, people seldom adopt new technology on faith alone.

THE EFFECT OF THE CRITICAL SUCCESS FACTORS (CSFs)

Each of the six critical success factors defines the speed through which an organization moves along the technology adoption curve. Unfortunately for the healthcare field, there has been very little successful information technology adoption that can be analyzed to provide empirical evidence or quantifiable results in order to be able to predict actual timelines and workload. Consequently, these CSFs often go unrecognized in healthcare, leading to poor information system design and development going forward.

The obvious question facing healthcare now is: How do we get out of this cycle of poor systems begetting more poor systems? Whether the information technology creates new functionality or replaces an existing system, an important point is that the outcomes resulting from the adoption must be measured and compared to previous statistics or results to illustrate the improvement (or not) from the new IT; ultimately, this change in outcomes must be communicated to the stakeholders. While all of this may seem extremely obvious, and perhaps even trivial, one of the fatal flaws that system designers often overlook is that new technology (regardless of its composition) requires an interface to human beings. If the stakeholders do not have their expectations properly established through effective communication right from the conception of the project, resistance to change and the other critical success factors may derail an otherwise very effective new technology application.

EXAMPLE STORY 1

Communication of expectations is the cornerstone of successful IT adoption.

Two teams of telephone pole installation technicians are hired to install telephone poles in a new residential subdivision. The existing crew is the best in the business and need very little guidance. A second crew is brand new, but they receive very little instruction as well – after all, they are only installing telephone poles (it's not like it's brain surgery!).

After the end of the first day, both teams report to their supervisor. When asked, the first team of experts reported that they had installed 25 poles that day – a new record for that area. When the supervisor asked the second crew team leader, he sheepishly replied that they had only installed two!

"Two? How can that be?" was the immediate retort from the boss. "Let's go out right now to see the work of the first team so that you can see how a real team does professional work!"

They all stormed out to the site in the subdivision where

the first team had worked. The supervisor looked proudly down the street – "See, that's championship work!"

To which the second team leader responded immediately – "Yeah, sure, but look how much of their poles is sticking out of the ground!"

Takeaways from the story:

- No matter how simple or straightforward it may appear to the user, the information system and technology request to the system developers is always new and complex. Therefore *no* instruction, clarification or detail should be considered too small to communicate. As we've all experienced from our own personal relationships, communication is the key to success.

GUIDELINES FOR SUCCESSFUL TECHNOLOGY ADOPTION

Why have we not been able to see the same successful technology development in healthcare that we have seen in many other industries to date?

The objective of this book is to highlight some of the key considerations that must be addressed when organizations adopt new technology, especially new information technology. These factors are consistent across industries and overlooking them has often led to the downfall of many IT initiatives in healthcare applications. Although being cognizant of them does not guarantee a successful implementation, it does increase the likelihood of a positive outcome.

The CSFs infer the following *conclusions* (in no direct order or relationship):

1. The objective of any new information system must be made clear at the beginning of the project so that everyone involved will know whether it's the creation of a new system or the revision of current functionality.

2. Technology performance and system outcome metrics must be established up-front so that the right controls are put in place at the outset – i.e., ongoing evaluation is paramount.

3. Of utmost import is the fact that all issues, both positives and negatives, related to the technology change must be, to the degree that they can be predicted, communicated effectively.

4. Every project, organization, person encounters both good luck and bad. At times, taking advantage of the good "bounces" is as critical as good strategic planning. Further, realizing that every project will have bad things happen is a first step in overcoming obstacles – which must be present or else the solution would have been created by now!

5. The reliance of IT as a cost saver must be abandoned (at least in the short term). New information systems have very seldom been implemented successfully when the benefits are limited solely to lowering costs.

This final conclusion (5) should be elaborated upon as it summarizes the entire theory and integrates it all (with conclusions 1, 2, 3 and 4) together. While it is quite true that many technology implementations are initially designed to address cost issues, these potential cost savings are often dwarfed by the onset of escalating costs pertaining to the implementation phase – once again, see Figure 1. Therefore, the project life is only sustained if there are other benefits to be gained – benefits that have to be measured objectively and in conjunction with the objectives stated in conclusion 1 – hence the need for the development of metrics in conclusion 2. This, of course, leads to the need for better documentation and communication of improvements (conclusion 3) and management of the unknown (conclusion 4) throughout the life of the project. If not, the technology initiative will die somewhere between Times 2 and 3 (on the technology adoption curve, Figure 1) as costs escalate – and the resistance to change movement will have claimed another victory for the status quo.

The bottom line is that change is necessary if we are to improve the way we do things. This is a very important consideration, as our healthcare system needs improvement. I am not advocating that we change the fundamental principles of the health system – just the operation of it. Currently, the present system is fraught with inefficiencies. Hospital departments and programs still cannot talk to each other electronically in most health organizations – let alone work together. One cannot access, in the curent year, in any simple and straightforward manner, which procedures have been delivered and the effectiveness of these procedures. We must begin to emphasize that any new initiative has to focus on developing a health information system in order to allow for information exchange among patients, government agencies, healthcare providers, educational institutions and private sector partners. It is hoped that the guidelines presented herein will assist in change management and increase the probability of future successful information system development and adoption.

Throughout the remainder of this book, I will refer to this technology adoption curve (Figure 1, page 27), as it will help us understand where the different industries were and how they overcame their obstacles to change. In addition, during the telling of the stories, I will step out of the stories in order to highlight an event or critical point – these sections will be *italicized* for ease of identification. I trust that these stories will allow all of us to view the healthcare issues from new perspectives.

Further, it must be noted that the six critical success factors (CSFs) that were discussed above (and proposed on page 24) are components of each of the stories presented. In detail, the first three CSFs (resistance to change, amount of training and stakeholder buy-in) relate to the role that I played as an educator and a change agent in each industry and are outlined in the section labeled "creating change." Next, the fourth CSF (consumer engagement) will be highlighted in the section entitled "the role of the consumer." The fifth CSF (ongoing performance reporting) is directly related to the creation and distribution of outcome metrics and will be discussed in the "performance measurement" section. The final CSF will be interspersed throughout the stories demonstrating confrontation relating to dealing with the unexpected. These stories, then, in addition to demonstrating new technology struggles from other industries, also assist in defining what is critical in overcoming the hurdles related to the adoption.

Finally, it must be reiterated that these are not the key factors necessary and sufficient to ensure a successful system implementation of any new technology. The task of identifying strategies for successful system development is quite complex and heavily dependent on the organization and the industry one is working within.

"Public participation in communicating with policy makers concerning the health care system is essential to closing the gaps in our health care system."

Dr. Robert Dugal,
Vice President, Policy, Planning and Research, Rx&D –
Canada's research-based Pharmaceutical Companies

❧

CHAPTER FOUR

The benefits of storytelling

What is the role of technology and computers in our society today? Who has access to them? Who is interested in having them? What is the point of putting health information (in electronic format) on the World Wide Web, if the people who need it most, the elderly, do not have access to it?

Undoubtedly, we've all heard these current questions. Further, we've heard comments like "people, mainly children, spend too much time in the home, isolated. Instead of getting together with their neighbours and friends, people are huddled away inside by themselves." Thus leading to the obvious conclusion: the Internet will be the end of the *community*, or perhaps our society, as we know it.

Oddly enough, these fears were not first expressed about computers or about children and their penchant for computer games and the Internet. These same comments were made centuries ago about books. After Gutenberg invented the printing press, information and knowledge became accessible to the masses. One no longer had to be privileged to learn. At first, as one would imagine, the demand for information and knowledge greatly surpassed the ability to satisfy it, thereby establishing a significant hunger for books. But soon, the demand and supply equalled out and factors stabilized.

The computer today has put everything, once again, out of balance. Newcomers to the Internet spend an inordinate amount of time in front of their computer. These newcomers exert much effort gathering information about things that they didn't even know they wanted information about (you may have to read this sentence a couple of times to assure yourself there is no typo!). Some scholars and columnists report that this is a bad thing. But how can that be? How can creating the desire to be inquisitive about new ideas be a bad thing? How can we be anything but further ahead if we have more information?

Most of us know that the next generation of managers – those born in the 1970s – has grown up with computers. Uploading, logging on, print drivers are all terms they use in their sleep (I know, they must have weird dreams!). Not surprising then that this generation employs computers the most. Demographic studies have shown that as family age decreases, and as income increases, the portion of households with computers rises. Computers are not a fad; they are critical to our growth. A computer, in and of itself, is not important because it doesn't know anything. It's simply a tool – a means to an end – a very expensive pencil, if you will. The computer is important, however, because it is, today, the best means of *getting* information.

We must not run away from computerization and the adoption of new technology. Yes, there are costs to making change, but these costs are worth it, because our most important societal right comes with it – our right to be educated. We should not merely accept new technology, we must demand it … and demand it now. Just like the banking customer who wants better service, we must demand better information. The next time your boss comments on an error in your judgment, just reply that it was the best you could do with the little information you had access to; if your boss wants better decisions, then tell him or her to give you the opportunity to access better information. Hopefully, your boss will respond by putting you on a user task force to define your information needs (all information systems can be improved) – and not fire you (after all, change does bring with it some inherent risks).

Great, but what does this have to do with storytelling? During the final stages of writing this book, I came across another very interesting book that I highly recommend. It's entitled *The Springboard: How Storytelling Ignites Action in Knowledge-Era Organizations* and was written by Stephen Denning (Butterworth-Heinemann, 2001). The author worked as Program Director of Knowledge Management at the World Bank in Washington, D.C. The book describes in great detail the issues relating to change and the massive resistance to change that exists across all segments of our society. It also illustrates how telling stories can help some people overcome this resistance by helping them see the positives about change, given other peoples' experiences. And this is what stories do – they help illuminate that the struggle is worthwhile.

Without truly being aware of it, I realized that I had constructed this book in the very same way. Instead of hitting the reader over the head with theories and ideas of why we need change (which I have done in the past), I decided to use my experience in other industries to illustrate not only the successes from other fields but the struggles as well. We get motivated by seeing other people's success, however we need to know it was not easy for them – that they had obstacles to overcome as well. Seeing that their obstacles were very similar is also beneficial as we gain ideas from their challenges – in many, many ways I have learned that misery really does love company!

In his book, Denning outlines many principles of storytelling – how to create the story (often very short in length; a page or two at most), key elements in the story and how to relate the story to others. The main point, I believe, is to make the story relevant in as many ways as possible so that the listener (or reader) can make the leap from the story to the issue at hand.

Throughout this book, I will attempt to draw parallels between the industries so that the stories can provide a connection. At the end of the book, I outline four very straightforward "prescriptions" that we must accomplish if we are to improve healthcare delivery. Each one of these industry examples will help point us all to these very specific objectives.

As an aside, if the concept of storytelling looks vaguely familiar to anyone who has attended business school, then it should because it is simply another form of teaching using the Case Study method. Pioneered by Harvard University, this methodology is used in almost all undergraduate and graduate business and management programs globally today (not necessarily exclusively, but as some part of the curriculum in a variety of courses). In a case study, the background is given so that the readers can immerse themselves in the particulars of the case. Then a problem is presented and the requirement is normally that of challenging the student to make the best decision(s) given the parameters that have been laid out. The cases can range in length from one paragraph to fifty pages or more. Whereas case studies require the reader to resolve the crisis, a story goes one step further by providing the resolution and then offers the connection between the situation and the outcome, thereby employing the story's issues or problems as powerful educational assistants. In this book, I will attempt to combine these two concepts into one (and use the name inter- changeably). My stories will vary in length (and hence detail) but will also be resolved so that the decisions and out- comes can be presented for illustrative purposes.

One story (or case study) relates to the healthcare industry but also cuts across many others – and this is "change and this phe- nomenon of the resistance to change." Why do people seem to object to a new idea before the words are even finished coming out of our mouths? We've all experienced it – some- times it may pertain to our work or maybe it relates to simple things in our lives – such as what side of the bed we sleep on with our partner. (If you don't believe me then just try it; go to bed tonight and without discussing it, lie down on the opposite side and see the reaction you get!) If we are to make change in the healthcare system, then we must overcome this resistance – be it by government, the Ministry of Health, bureaucrats, doctors or even other patients; we must not let this change management issue detract us from our objectives.

EXAMPLE STORY 2

Why is Change Management so important?

In a large Academic Health Science Centre around the mid-1990s, the diagnostic imaging department was going through the final stages of the conversion to a completely film-less radiology process – in other words, moving to electronic images of x-rays and the like. During this conversion, the doctors were notified and then sent their patients' images by emails. By late morning of the first day of the transition, many doctors complained that they had yet to receive their patients' x-ray results. Apparently, the doctors did not check their emails.

In an effort to ensure the success of the conversion, the imaging department then began to send the doctors the radiology results on a computer diskette or compact disks (CD-ROM, depending on the size of the file). Unfortunately, the doctors still continued to complain about the tardiness of the results. Even though they received the diskettes and CDs in a timely manner, they could <u>not</u> match the arrival of these hardware supplies to their own information needs. This is not to say that the physicians were not computer literate, but rather inexperienced at identifying the connection between CDs and patient x-rays. So the imaging department hit upon a great idea: they continued to used the CDs but now sent them to the doctors via internal hospital delivery system in the traditional large x-ray envelopes. Recognizing the envelopes, the doctors opened them immediately, placed the CDs in their computers and started reviewing the results.

Takeaways from the story:

- This story is a great illustration of the need to make the link (perhaps through education or training) between the new technology and the old ways of doing things. It's worth noting that the adoption was not quite complete, however, until the final functionality was arrived at: the quality of the image had to be as good or better than what they had ... or else the adoption would never have taken place, no matter how easily the results were accessed.

Quite simply, people hate change. You may think this is an obvious remark or even an overstatement. When it comes to evolving technology, however, the need to focus on people's acceptance to change cannot be overstated. But why? Well, it really comes down to a very basic phenomenon – fight for survival, or at least the perception of it. You see, when change happens, people who do not adjust their work patterns begin to fail. They fail because the old ways of doing things do not work within the new system. Soon their failures mount and more bad things happen.

The people that do succeed are the ones who first realize that the way they did things before was not perfect and that new technology has allowed them to improve. Once they have accepted the change, they begin to operate more efficiently and effectively than they ever did before. This is a very important point: if you operate the exact same way after the introduction of new technology as you did before the introduction, then you have missed a great opportunity to improve your processes and your outcomes. Change is not about getting a new computer – change is about how you are going to take advantage of it. This requires work as well as the important realization that the way you have always done things can, and must, be improved. Furthermore, effective change management requires time; hence, throughout the healthcare system, one of our first requirements is the "prescription for patience."

"Health care in the 21st century must be patient-centered, consumer-driven and provider-friendly."

Bill Frist,
Senate Majority Leader, United States Senate,
Washington, DC.

⚜

CHAPTER FIVE

The stories:
my experience and perspective

In this chapter, I provide three stories from three industries that will demonstrate the six critical success factors and how they relate to the adoption of new technology. In order to assist with the storytelling, I will step out of the stories at certain points and describe the impact that these specific points have on healthcare and its own technology adoption; these commentaries will be illustrated by *italics*.

I believe that many of the people who have been very successful (perhaps measured by great leaps in personal wealth) in the last two decades or so have been the people who have made fantastic strides in innovating technology – people like Bill Gates of Microsoft, among others. It is my opinion that, in the next decade, the truly successful people will be the ones who can take this recent surge of technological advancement and apply it to new areas. Many businesses and other organizations have been overwhelmed with the technological breakthroughs of the last ten to twenty years. Only a very small percentage, however, have been able to capitalize on all of these developments and integrate them into daily operations. These few are the ones that are now getting ahead of their competition. And this opportunity for competitive advantage will continue to be ripe for exploitation until all of us are on the same playing field once more. Based on my observations, however, and the wide disparity in penchant that individuals and organizations have toward technology, we may never have an even playing field again. The growth in the technology industry is so rapid that the number of options and combinations of innovation and creativity is virtually limitless.

In order to capitalize on these circumstances (as opposed to being continually frustrated), I have concentrated my own professional career on bringing innovation as well as new technologies and ideas to different areas. Further, in my opinion, these opportunities are plentiful. So plentiful in fact that I have been able to pick and choose any ones I wanted. So I picked the areas that I enjoyed most – corporate and consumer banking, post-secondary education, sports and healthcare. It may sound like an odd mix, and it is, but I am passionate about them all and that's what really counts.

The majority of people, and businesses themselves for that matter, are so busy with their day-to-day lives, that they cannot see or cannot afford the time to learn how to make their lives and jobs easier. In other words, they get caught up in a working harder cycle rather thanworking smarter. When a deadline approaches, instead of taking the time to think about how best to do the task, they stay with the same processes that got them behind in the first place, except now they work twice as hard. This hard work gets reinforced in the short run and the next time, the staff works even harder – the cycle continues until they hit the limit and the system fails completely! Success requires creative thinking.

As a result, since people do not budget enough time in their schedules for "creative thinking," they need someone to help them, or as we say in the academic literature they need a change agent, someone who can assist in designing working smarter solutions. This agent then is seen as the champion to help make all the necessary adjustments. What is beautiful about all of this is the "halo effect." Once you've made a significant impact in one area, people believe that you can make the same advancements in others, and they keep coming to you for advice. And then the opportunities just keep multiplying. The first section is about one of these applications: an application of contemporary state-of-the-art computer technology to the world of banking and credit. The two subsequent sections provide the education and the professional hockey (National Hockey League or NHL) stories, respectively.

THE BANKING STORY

In this section, we focus on a fairly new discipline (started within the last half-century) which very few people are even cognizant about – that is, credit scoring. Simply put, credit scoring is the study of the statistical relationships between the data contained on the application for credit and the outcome of this credit extension (in other words, whether someone turned out to be a good/profitable or a bad/delinquent customer). Very briefly, information that you enter on an application form for a credit card, let's say, is analyzed and your information (or answers to questions such as income, time on job) is then entered into a model. The result of this model, or mathematical equation, is called a score (hence the term "credit scoring") and this score is compared to a minimum score called a "cut-off score." If your (or any applicant's) score is above the minimum, then the application is approved and the credit is extended. If not, the application for credit is denied.

As with the other stories that follow, in the first subsection we will examine how this new information system (and the new technology required) created change and affected the decision-makers in the industry. Following, I will present the major effect that consumers have had on the industry in the United States and in Canada. The final subsection of this story will present further discussion on performance measurement and how this will drive the industry in the next decade.

Creating change

Credit scoring models were first developed for consumer credit. Based on the statistical analyses of historical data, certain financial variables or indicators are determined to be important in the evaluation process of the potential new consumer's financial stability and strength. Hence, the result is a predictive relationship between the answers on an application form for credit and the likelihood of the customer paying the obligation (being good) or not (going delinquent). This relationship is called a "statistical model" or a "credit scorecard."

*Applying statistical methods to the credit decision has been extremely successful. In particular, the area of credit scoring for consumer credit has developed into a multi-million dollar industry. But how did this happen? How was this industry so successful in adopting new technology where other industries have been much more reluctant? In fact, credit scoring was **not** accepted at first as a panacea that was going to cure all in the risk management area of the banks. However, over time the concept took hold to the point where today just* *about every credit granting institution in North America uses some form of scoring. The history is to follow.*

The development, implementation and acceptance of scoring over time from management personnel at banks and credit card companies can be best described as a progression through three phases. Phase 1, the Denial Phase, involves the rejection of the whole principle of using statistics to adjudicate credit. What's wrong with the old way? It's worked up until now, why change it? What do statistics have to do with credit evaluation? In the end the objection is one of removing the decision making from solely the credit manager's purview to one where the manager is being assisted by a model, or a decision support system (DSS). If the manager then does not agree with the model's recommendation (either to approve or decline the credit application) then it is categorized as an "override." These overrides are a very sensitive topic as they are measured and tracked with the manager being responsible to justify the case when too many occur. As a scorecard developer in the mid-1980s, the question that I heard most was: "How can this new technology replace all of the experience that rests in the human resources of the credit lender?"

The most effective way of addressing this objection is to illustrate the benefits of scoring – both those that are possible and those that have been experienced by other financial institutions (including the competition). This will allow a certain comfort level to, at the very least, give scoring an opportunity to exhibit benefits during a trial period (and hopefully reach Time 4 on the technology adoption curve.

Phase 2, the Acceptance Phase, involves the total acceptance of scoring. It works! Here, most credit managers begin to show blind faith in the modelling process because of the benefits that have been experienced first-hand. Further, there is a feeling that there is no need for scorecard monitoring and constant re-evaluation.

> *The best way to address this problem is to keep on top of the training issues and reinforce the basic theory – stressing both the advantages and shortcomings of this new technology. In this way, managers are constantly reminded of the pitfall of relying too heavily on the scorecards. Some observers in this industry have remarked that this phase is more dangerous than Phase 1 because technology has been implemented but is not truly being managed. We will return to this observation in the later section on the healthcare industry.*

Phase 3, the Maturation Phase, involves the realization that scoring models are tools – very effective tools – but nonetheless, just tools. To get the most out of these tools, the scoring models must be properly integrated into the strategic objectives of the portfolio. At this point, scoring is not seen as a separate entity, but rather as a single, very important component in the adjudication process.

> *Once the success of credit scoring spread, new features began to be developed in order to try and obtain the benefits of scoring faster and with more accuracy. Application processing software was introduced and the human interface (i.e., the credit manager) was, in some places, removed from the credit evaluation process altogether. In some detail, appli-*

*cation data can now be entered into an automated processing unit through the use of dedicated software. The score is then automatically generated and a credit decision is made without any internal or external review. In some institutions, a third party processor (separate organization whose sole function is computerized credit scoring) is contracted to handle all of the application scoring and processing details. This then takes advantage of all the efficiencies offered by scoring. In short, it is possible to apply for credit, have it approved and the credit card or account opened **without any human interaction** during the entire process.*

Supportive organizations

As stated, virtually every bank and trust company in North America currently employs some form of credit scoring. Unfortunately, due to the technical sophistication of the statistical analysis involved in the creation and implementation of scoring models, there has been a scarcity of resources to turn to for adequate training and research. This prompted the need for the creation of an association that would address these training and implementation issues that continually arise within the credit scoring community – this would be the first of its kind in the world. Consequently, in June 1992, the CSRSA (Credit Scoring and Risk Strategy Association, www.CSRSA.com) was formed and I became the founding president. This association, more than anything else, over the years has become a good sounding board where member institutions meet and discuss with others in the industry. This sharing of information has proven to be very beneficial due to the fact that scoring problems (and solutions) are often shared by all credit organizations.

The need for this type of association became quite evident during the early 1990s when I was working with a number of bank managers. They didn't really care how the scorecards were built or even the statistics behind the development of their own tools (this was hard for me to understand!). However, they did have many questions about how to use the scorecards (and manage them) and there was nowhere to turn. (Scorecard developers spend most of their resources building models and demonstrating little desire to support them.) Therefore, with very little training support and buy-in opportunity, it's no wonder the adoption of this technology was slow to occur at first (see Phase 1 discussion above).

In order to fill this void, at one bank we sent out repeated messages to our branch associates to update them on the conversion and provide a presence of such support both technical and strategic. In one instance, along with the regular memorandum, the bank sent out a "coffee cup coaster" that, in an effort to be creative, was shaped exactly like a three-and-a-quarter-inch diskette. This coaster was made with plastic on one side and a soft felt-like material on the other so that cups and glasses would not slide. In addition, there was writing on the coaster giving some quick helpful hints to ensure effective navigation through the new credit scoring technology with as little problem as possible.

A few days after the package went out, the technical call centre received a number of irate calls demanding how to get the "diskette cleaner" out of their floppy drive! Obviously there was a need for some training material to outline the details of the training material. The loan associates automatically thought the diskette-like coaster should go into the diskette drive (a quite natural assumption, actually) and never really read the instructions that came with it. Since it was made to look like a computer diskette, they immediately put it into the floppy drive. Unfortunately, it was flexible and comprised of soft material and the drive could not eject it (obviously a true floppy disk). In the end, many computers had to be manually serviced to get the floppy coasters out!

Takeaways from the story

- No one industry has the monopoly on early adopters and no one industry is comprised of only people that resist change. All industries face the exact same challenges. They address them in different ways and there are different outcomes, but in the end, the problems are the same. That is the message in this book: We must be able to learn from other industries in order to save healthcare from the same "growing pains" and mistakes that other industries have already experienced, learned from and then progressed. To this end, let's now examine this industry's adoption of new technology with respect to the first three of our six critical success factors.

1. Amount of industry experience in using technology

The banking, and more specifically, the credit industry has had a fairly long history of using technology to its advantage. This experience has allowed it to flourish when many other industries are still struggling. It's important to emphasize that this experience can only be gained over time – and that is the biggest investment that the banking industry has made. They invested in technology so long ago that they have created a culture where technology is not viewed as change but as the status quo. If we look back only a quarter-century ago, we had to get to our branch of the bank in order to access funds. Now twenty-five years later, we can deposit a cheque and access funds anywhere in the world at any time. We can dial-in and make payments for bills or move money between accounts. Often payroll is deposited directly into the bank of our own designation (i.e., direct deposit) making a trip to our own bank a requirement of the past. As a result, this experience has created an environment of belief that technology can improve business operations and exceed expectations.

2. Amount of training both before and during the transition

The credit industry has recognized the value-add that training can provide. First, many scorecard developers and industry consultants now have regular training initiatives all over the world. Second, there is a continuing stream of credit scoring conferences worldwide that presents the latest research and technology advancement so that customers are aware of the state-of-the-art. Lastly, credit risk managers have created associations to ensure that the proper support and training would always be available.

3. Amount of buy-in (or contribution during design) from the different stakeholder groups

In the early years, there was a lot of resistance to credit scoring. Bank managers and loan officers felt that their knowledge could not be replicated by a computer model. There was no way that a model could capture all of the years of experience and the subjectivity that goes into the art of making credit decisions. This resistance permeated the industry for quite a long time (and still does today if we examine certain areas such as small business scoring) until the results revealed the benefits of scoring: improved bottom line effects. Most models today are not created in spite of the managers but rather include them as critical elements of the design and development of these tools. This involvement insures better models and more buy-in. The loan officers are aware of the trade-offs and limitations inherent in the model building process such that they can not only use but also defend the model. This is critical to long-term industry adoption and credit scoring's success.

The role of the consumer

Since every major financial institution in North America currently employs some form of credit scoring, all of us have been credit scored at one point or another. Yet, the average consumer has very little knowledge of its existence, let alone what constitutes the score and how well he or she performs with respect to everyone else. As we have learned from other industries, this will change dramatically over the next decade.

Let's first examine the banking industry and the effect of consumerism over the last twenty-five years. We no longer live in a time where people are satisfied to get their cash in person from only one branch of one bank between the hours of 10am and 3pm, Monday through Friday. It was not that long ago that going to your own branch was the only way to obtain cash. If I had approached my father back then and said: "Dad, I have a dream, a dream that someday people will be lining up to get cash from a wall," I wonder what his response would have been. He probably would not have let me out of the house ever again … and he hardly let me out as it was. It's a good thing I never said that. If I had, however, I would have been correct.

The move to new automated teller machines (ATM) technology, however, was not a smooth process for the banks at the beginning. The amount of work required to manage the transition was not insignificant. First, there was the need for additional personnel to guide the customers to the ATMs (while still maintaining the teller staff). In effect, they were running and supporting two systems in parallel. More importantly, however, they employed an innovative strategy that turned out to be one of the main reasons for the successful technology adoption – they *chose* to actually drive the workload up. In effect, in the early 1990s, the banks increased rather than decreased the number of hours they were open. Banks stayed open late during the week and often on Saturdays and some even on Sundays. This then helped stir up demand for more services (that the banks would then fulfil) and also raised customer expectations. Customers began to get used to doing their banking at times when it was convenient for them rather than having to take time off work to meet with the branch manager.

Over time, these expectations and services migrated to an electronic medium for delivery resulting in bank hours returning to what they had been in the late eighties. In fact, very few bank branches are open past 6pm or on weekends any more. It's only now that the banks are reaping the reward of less work and higher customer satisfaction through better technology (we are well beyond Time 4 on the technology adoption curve).

Some customers resisted and still today have not converted, however, they are very much in the minority. Others took many years, gradually adopting the ATMs one feature at a time, usually starting with withdrawing cash and then escalating their use to include depositing cheques, paying bills and so on. Part of the reason for the resistance was the amount of perceived work involved in learning a new system (in addition to the basic urge to resist change).

When people started using ATMs to withdraw cash, they would count their money (as always) and if the amount was not correct on first count, the immediate assumption was that the machine was wrong and now they would have to fight with someone to get it fixed – more work! Nowadays, if the count is not correct, we recount it with the expectations that the ATM was right and that we counted incorrectly. Why? Expectations, based on experience, have led us to believe that the machine is not wrong (after years of being accurate), that we have counted wrong, or two bills are stuck together, or some other explanation. The expectation of more work has been eliminated due to our experiences.

In addition, another reason for early resistance was that many consumers felt it was not a decision or choice they were making but one that was being made for them by the banks, thereby resisting the imposition.

Finally, because there was little experience using this type of technology effectively (or perhaps any type of computers) at that time, there was no buy-in on behalf of the public and little perceived benefit. It was only through the banks' relentless commitment to ATMs that the public finally started to see the benefits of being able to access cash from anywhere at any time and the ability to do most of their banking from their home over the phone line or on the Web. Today, the consumers are the ones driving the change, requesting the ability to apply for a mortgage or car loan via the Internet (remember the best line that a systems developer can hear: Can you get the system to do this?). Today, it's possible to log on at midnight from home, apply for a line of credit and receive an email the next morning confirming not only that the bank received the application but also confirming the approval of the request and the access to funds, all features driven by consumer acceptance of technology and demanded by the power of consumerism as a whole.

> *It's interesting to note that the move through the early stages of the technology adoption curve (Figure 1, page 27; Time 0 to 3) in banking was supported by the fact that banking customers had no option and had to learn the technology if they wanted to access their funds at any time, from anywhere. This uniqueness gave the technology time to make a difference and illustrate the benefits. (It should be noted that banks still allow their customers to use tellers if they so choose.)*

Returning to credit, very few of us, and less and less each year, can avoid using credit. In today's economy, having established credit in itself is a measure of creditworthiness. In my parents' generation, having a credit card had a stigma attached to it: "Only those that cannot afford to pay for it use credit!" Applying for credit (other than for a mortgage) was perceived as a sign of bad financial management. For the longest time, my father's only credit card was a gas company card and was to be used only for vacations and then, *only* for emergencies (like the time our muffler system fell off the car while driving in the US and we had to get it repaired; the use of credit in that situation was a "no-brainer"). Today, most consumers have multiple credit cards available to them in their wallets and purses.

Unfortunately, very few customers know much about managing credit effectively and what comprises the basic mechanics. Sure, we all know that paying bills is good and not paying them is bad, but beyond that it's a mystery. However, we should know more and we can use the scoring methodology to help us.

There are two main credit bureaus in Canada (Trans Union and Equifax) and three in the US (these two plus Experian); they all retain information on all credit consumers in the country for a maximum period of seven years. (Therefore, a missed payment from ten years ago will no longer show on file.) Every one of us should check our credit bureau file once a year or so to make sure that the content is accurate. You can access information about getting a copy of your file through the Internet as well as directly with both bureaus that have customer service departments that deal with complaints or inaccuracies. The mere fact that these databases exist and they contain data on you should be reason enough to want to check the veracity of the data. However, there is a more critical reason: every time that you apply for credit in the future, the credit granter will check the bureaus (usually one or the other, but sometimes both) for information before your application is approved. If there exists an error in your file, your application could get turned down; by the time you get the error rectified, you may have missed the opportunity to purchase a home or lost the chance to take advantage of whatever it was you wanted the credit for in the first place.

Why is credit scoring important if I am just checking the accuracy of data in my credit file? Technology brings with it advantages in three areas: efficiency, effectiveness and consistency. We have discussed the first two at length, but here we will address consistency. One of the main reasons to move to quantitative type decision support (such as a score) is to remove a lot of the subjectivity that exists in making decisions, which can lead to misinterpretation of the facts and the inclusion of any inherent bias (within the system or even within the decision-maker). With a score, it does not matter who is making the decision, it will always be the same because the scorecard is the same for each credit officer. Hence, there is consistency in decision-making. As a result, when a group of customers are scored, one can easily rank-order the entire group by risk. In other words, a consumer could examine their file and be in the dark as to whether they have a good file or a bad file (assuming that the file is error-free) with respect to the public at large.

With a credit score, and knowledge of the score distribution for the population, consumers can know precisely how they stack up and what percentile they are in with respect to everyone else. So, if you find that your score places you in the top ten percent of the population regarding credit risk, then you know that you should be able to be approved for just about any credit product that you can afford (subject to income and so on). If you are in the bottom ten percent, for example, then you know that you should start learning more about managing your credit, because the likelihood of being approved for any new credit vehicle in the immediate future is very low. (There are some creditors who are looking for people who have low scores so as to capitalize on the fact that they would have very little credit option – in exchange for this, of course, they will often charge a much higher interest rate to cover their increased risk. Either way, the options are very few if your credit profile is poor!) Hence, we should all know how we rank and how to improve our standing and/or correct errors or omissions.

To date, there has been very little usage of credit scores by the public in Canada. In the United States, however, the credit market is much more mature. First of all, credit card portfolios and banks have the ability to access a consumer's credit bureau file without the consumer's consent (this is not possible in Canada). Therefore, a bank in the US can use a credit bureau score to rate people's risk and then send out a pre-approved credit application to all customers that are over a certain risk level (without first consulting the consumer). Consequently, consumers who have managed their previous credit well (which is the basis for a credit score) will be inundated with these credit solicitations from a never-ending stream of organizations. This proliferation of credit offerings has consequently made the public more aware of credit bureaus as a result and they're much more savvy about managing their overall credit profile.

4. Level of consumer (or end-user) influence during early stages of adoption

Public awareness in the US population has led consumers to demand access to their credit score (and not just their credit bureau file or raw data). They can access a number of different sites (such as myfico.com) to find out their score. There is a feature that offers a simulation exercise or game where the consumer can even vary some of their data to see if their score will improve or not. (*This helps the consumer understand the effect of making payments on time and the negative implications of skipping regular payments.*) The result is that consumers are educating themselves about credit and a more educated consumer leads to better self-selection of customers (people will not apply for things they cannot possibly afford – if not, the

Mercedes dealership would be swamped every day with people applying and being turned down). Better educated and higher quality customers (as a whole) then lead to lower bad debt and loan losses and, ultimately, to lower interest rates – which is good for the economy!

In the end, in Canada, the public needs to be more knowledgeable about credit and credit scores, similar to the consuming public in the US. This will lead to a better educated consumer who will drive change just as on the banking and deposit side. On top of everything else already noted, this information will empower the consumer to make better decisions and behave more responsibly. How can more information and better education ever be considered a bad thing?

Performance measurement

The story of banking and credit scoring as an example of successful technology adoption is so strong that there are many lessons to be learned. Here, we will describe the role that performance measurement had in expediting the adoption of this technology over time.

Most credit scorecards are built to address the good/bad (or profitable/delinquent) decision. Financial institutions are interested in what makes a good loan and what is indicative of a more risky loan (possibly bad). In order to build a scorecard that rank orders individuals based on the odds of being a good or a bad customer, one must first define very specifically these two principal sets. A good account is an account that has, for the most part, paid their financial obligations in full and on time. A good account is not necessarily an account that has never been delinquent. There are times when accounts go into arrears for a brief period of time (one cycle late) over a long evaluation period and this account should still be classified as a good. This is due to the fact that, as a whole, the customer has exhibited good payment behaviour. Basically, the rule of thumb for a good account is – if the lender had to do it over again they would.

Contrarily, a bad account is an account that if the lender had the opportunity to do it over they would not. This is an account that typically has been delinquent many times during a short time period; or perhaps is an account that is currently 90 days past due or worse. Also, accounts that have been put into a non-performing category or have been written-off are classified as bads – these are, in fact, the worst of all the bads. It's important to note, however, that a bad is not necessarily an account that has been written-off or put into collections. Some bads are just accounts that have been such a nuisance that it costs more to keep them current than the revenue gained from interest charges and late fees.

A cut-off score can be effectively established in one of two ways. First, since a scorecard rank orders all applicants by risk (the documentation accompanying the scorecard at completion of analysis provides detailed information concerning the score breakdown of the development sample), a cut-off score can be set by referring to the cumulative statistics in an attempt to match previous acceptance rates. Then if we wish to accept (say) 70% of all applicants in the future, a cut-off score is set at the 30th percentile – we expect 70% of all applicants to score at or above this score.

A second method for cut-off score establishment involves the calculation of a breakeven score. This requires a fairly good estimate of the number of goods (revenue generation) it takes to cover the losses from one bad – often in the range of 5 to 1 (i.e., the revenue from 5 goods roughly approximates the loss from a single bad). If this is true, then the cut-off score should be set at the score equivalent to an odds quote of 5 to 1. In this way, at the margin, we are breaking even for all accounts in the score range at the cut-off. Any accounts booked above this score will be profit generating, on average. Remember, the scorecard rank orders by risk – therefore, higher scores relate to higher probability of good, or more profitable, accounts as a whole.

Outcome measurement

Once scorecard development has been completed, the task turns to trying to get the banks, for instance, to adopt it. This is done by preparing a business case: this consists of weighing the cost of the scores against the benefit of either potential revenue (from a new account that would not otherwise be approved) or increased collections (from working accounts that may not have otherwise been identified as lucrative). The difficult thing in this situation is having a consensus as to what the potential revenue is for an additional account or being able to state with any accuracy that that account would not have been booked without the new technology. However the credit industry is in such a mature state that information systems (dedicated to monitoring credit scoring outcomes) have been built that allow for research to take place during the course of normal operations. (*This is a great example of how technology itself can make the case for its own adoption.*)

For example, if the research question is to determine whether or not a credit bureau scorecard can improve bottom line profits (i.e., increased collections outweigh the costs), we can illustrate the benefits in a few different ways:

- An improvement of dollars collected for equivalent number of accounts worked (e.g., $1.9 million at the 40% mark)
- A reduction in bureau files requested and scored (only require scores on delinquent accounts rather than the whole portfolio)
- An increase in the frequency of obtaining bureau scores (due to lower costs and increased collections, the score can be purchased every month).

This then provides a platform for discussing the fourth and fifth CSF.

5. Level of effective reporting on the status of the outcome measures during and post implementation

One of the big accomplishments that this industry has made over the last couple of decades is acceptance of standards for performance measurement. The comparison of loan losses to the cost per account scored is recognized and accepted as a standard business case to move ahead to new scoring technologies. Should the cost of buying and implementing the scores be less than the expected benefit from its utilization (in reducing loan losses), then the resistance to employing the new technology decreases with innovation being the biggest winner.

6. Level of effectiveness in dealing with good or bad fortune

There is really no way to plan for, or rely on, unforeseen circumstances, however, we all know that they must exist. The measure of success of an initiative or program is learning to deal with either good or bad luck in the most positive manner possible. When credit scoring was first introduced, the decision process surrounding credit extension was in its infancy and hence, very disorganized. Even though there was a creditability gap between vendors and the industry regarding the potential of scoring to reduce loan losses, there was definitely a mutually accepted need to implement some consistency. In a sense, the *consistency* objective helped scoring buy time to show the industry how well it would improve efficiency (reduce time and cost of making the credit decision) and effectiveness (lower loan losses).

THE EDUCATION STORY

In the fall of 1997, a team of faculty members from the Department of Health Policy, Management and Evaluation (HPME, University of Toronto) began work on the introduction of Distance Education Technology (DET) into the Masters of Health Administration (MHA/MHSc) course curriculum. This is their story.

The Department of HPME (formerly, the Department of Health Administration) has had a long and successful history, which recently celebrated its fiftieth anniversary. One of the main strengths of the Department, and the educational programs that it offers, is that it has been able to grow and adapt to meet the changing needs of its target population – namely health professionals. These educational programs have evolved from a single diploma program in early years to the delivery of two Masters programs (MHSc for professionals and MSc with a research focus) and a Doctoral program which, up until the mid-1990s, were offered in very traditional on-campus, full-time formats.

In the most recent years, a number of factors forced the Department to consider changes once again. First, the competition for graduate students, both internal and external to the University, has increased substantially. Many business school Master of Business Administration (MBA) programs, for instance, began soliciting healthcare managers emphasizing the benefit of a more general Administration degree. Second, the "business school" option became more attractive with Executive MBA programs and one-year master's programs. Third, the evolution of Distance Master's programs offered by many types of Administration programs further expanded the Department's competition from the greater Toronto area to virtually worldwide. Finally, the economic recession of the early 1990s made it much more difficult to attract future students – both in quality and in numbers – due to the fact that fewer and fewer potential students could afford to, or could risk to take two years off work to complete the curriculum.

Creating change

As a result, in the fall of 1994, the Department of Health Administration decided to change the professional Master's program from a traditional two-year format to a modular "executive" type format where students would meet only once every three (sometimes four) weeks for intensive on-campus course work. (In effect, students are on campus normally five times a semester, called Blocks, where each Block starts on Wednesday evening, and continues all day Thursday, Friday and Saturday.) This change allowed the incoming students to keep their full-time jobs as well as maintain other commitments while studying for a Master's degree – which could be completed in less than two years (approximately 20 months).

Consequently, the Department began creatively targeting new types of full-time students. This targeting was done through the attractive nature of the innovative modular structure and by considering students who did not necessarily reside in downtown Toronto. Since students were no longer required to be on campus every day or even every week, it became quite conceivable that students could either drive or fly into Toronto once a month. It became evident, as a result, that there would need to be contact at a distance with these students, who would not be on campus, from this time forward, the vast majority of time. Computer technology was seen as the vehicle to provide this contact.

Without the move to an electronic communication environment, the Department would have had to rely much more on mail (the old-fashion kind), faxes and courier services – all of which suffer in comparison to the technological alternatives. In the traditional on-campus full-time format, classes would be held once (and sometimes, twice) a week. In this scenario, the communication between students and faculty (regarding both course work and administrative issues) was very straightforward. In the off-campus, modular structure, interaction between the Department and the students would be strained using old communication media. For instance, updates to course work would have to be faxed, mailed or telephoned – options which would not be optimal due to the fact that they are costly and very time consuming.

Over the first three years of the modular format, from the fall of 1994 through to the summer of 1997, the Department began to migrate to newer forms of electronic communication technology. This migration was very informal and, consequently, lacked an overall strategic plan. For example, not unlike other university and college programs, electronic mail (e-mail) had been adopted and encouraged by the Department during this time frame. Further, through the use of mailing lists (listservs) and the Department Web site, students were presented with the opportunity to avail themselves of one-to-many and many-to-many modes of communication. However, the students did not embrace these new technologies, even though they have been proven to be effective in many other academic settings. Part of the explanation from the students was that they felt there was an inconsistent message sent to them from the Department and the faculty members due to incomplete and sporadic usage across the faculty and the courses.

*This inconsistent adoption by faculty (and widespread resistance to change) led to the actual **lack of technology adoption** that was taking place on the part of the students. For instance, an informal poll of second year students revealed that they had never used two of the newer communication media (the listservs and the Web page). In fact, many relied on other group members, perhaps those who were less reticent about technology, to read e-mail and listserv notices. These technically sophisticated students would then physically distribute the notes or information to the group (through faxes and/or voice mail). Previously, some faculty members had posted course notes on the Internet thinking that students would download the files electronically from the Department Web site – unfortunately, they were, in fact, getting hard copies (i.e., printed) from secre-*

taries and photocopying them for themselves and their class-mates. Students, even in a new era of the Internet (with information at the fingertips) and an innovative, executive-type teaching format, were still relying on old forms of communication.

Consequently, in the fall of 1997, two facts became evident. First, the Department needed to develop an information systems plan for electronic course support complete with timetables. This would then produce a consistent message to the students in addition to creating a mechanism for feedback should the adoption run into hurdles. Second, unless the students could see the benefits from changing to newer communication media (and that these benefits outweighed the perceived costs), they would be very resistant to embracing the newer technology.

Unfortunately, users often do not know what information would be useful. If they did, then they would have generated the information long ago. In management theory, much has been written concerning the ability of managers to identify their information needs. This is a very difficult task, and many approaches have been tested to accomplish this feat – with varying degrees of success.

On the first day of class, once the students had been informed that we were going ahead with the introduction of Distance Education Technology (DET), the reaction was explosive. Their main complaint centred on the idea of being forced to learn new technology with little or no benefits. Even though the students themselves agreed that the objectives and subsequent benefits listed above were worthwhile pursuing, the relationship between DET and achieving these goals was not evident. However, the initial feedback from the students notwith-standing, we were able to convince the students to introduce DET into the course on one principle: the students recognized that improvement in course communication was needed and that we had to begin to investigate options for future students. This consideration was much more influential in getting the students to agree to the exercise than positioning the use of the technology to help them with their problems this year.

In short, the student resistance to the DET related to two factors: (i) there was non-trivial work associated with learning DET; and (ii) the relationship between their stated objectives and the DET was not apparent. Ultimately, the benefits became inconsequential compared to the perceived associated costs (i.e., learning curve time).

> *We attempted to assure them that technology itself has sim-plified the adoption process but they were still reluctant to go forth, insisting that they had little computer knowledge. It was only with time and constant support that the students started to become more comfortable with the software, with making mistakes and with their current computer skills.*

Takeaways from the story

- Although it took approximately three years, the depart-ment has eventually reached a point where the students have come to see the benefits that DET can offer. Further, there is realization that these benefits actually out-weigh the cost of time that must be invested *before* the technology can be implemented.

This was achieved on an incremental basis by adhering to the following process:

- expose the students to the technology outlining the benefits to their learning objectives
- train students on the operational mechanics of DET as close to the start of the term as possible
- carefully select early adopters (keen faculty with courses that lend themselves well to technology and/or change issues)
- implement the DET in these selected pilot courses
- fully immerse the students by motivating them (on-line and almost immediate access to grades).

This final step of the full student immersion cannot be overstated. The students at many times wanted to back out of using the technology – due to computer glitches and downtime. If we had acquiesced, then we may never have progressed to where we are today. By forcing the students to work through the problems, they not only see the true benefits of DET, but they are better suited to handle innovation in the future – as there is no technology innovation without frustration. (This is very reminiscent of the banking scenario where clients were ultimately forced to interact with new technology.) We have now moved from a student environment of *aggressive ignorance* (i.e., I don't want to have to learn something else) to one where the students are adamant about pushing change into the program.

In summary, it's important to emphasize to all of the stakeholders, as the transition to DET is taking place, that the objective was not to replace student-faculty interaction, but rather to enhance it. If the technology can be seen to support communication in the changing academic environment, then it will be better received. If it is seen, however, as solely a replacement for current forms of communication, then it is less likely to be accepted.

One way of highlighting the innovation was to provide students functionality that did not previously exist – such as allowing the students to access their grades online throughout the term. Their grades were available three days at most after their assignments had been submitted, where historically it could take up to three weeks to get graded feedback. This quick turnaround fostered a more trusting environment and illustrated to the students how DET could address a high priority information need – "How well am I doing?" One student comment emphasized this point: "The use of incentives is a strategy for achieving buy-in from the learners and increasing the utilization of the software. For example, encouraging students to access grades for assignments through the system and to submit assignments using [DET] are two ideas that were successful in the [Management] Information Systems course."

In terms of the six critical success factors of technology adoption (Figure 1, page 27), what are the reasons for a rather successful implementation in this story?

1. Amount of industry experience in using technology
Clearly the students have much more sophistication regarding technology than "customers" in other industries due to their age, education, information needs and overall life experience. Even though the students were reluctant to admit, or perhaps recognize, the significance of this experience (gained from many industries including education), it did help expedite the

passage through the early parts of the technology adoption curve (Times 0 through 3).

2. Amount of training both before and during the transition

Our experience in the first year reinforced the fact that students required specific DET training. Moreover, this training should occur as close to the time as when they start using the DET as possible. This need for training has been consistently documented in recent literature concerning Web-based course tools. As well, the relationship between the career learning objectives and the DET must be highlighted (i.e., Why are we doing this?). This relationship should not be assumed to be readily apparent. Today, students and lecturers receive training and this training is held as close to the start of the semester as possible.

In addition to the actual training on the software itself, there were educational sessions detailing what the benefits of the system would be. In this way, there would be a link between some of their previously stated objectives and the implementation of the software. Otherwise, we run the risk of the link being overlooked (no matter how obvious it is to the system developers) and then the system may appear to be change just for the sake of change.

3. Amount of buy-in (or contribution during design) from the different stakeholder groups

I have taught this MIS-type course many times over the last decade to many different groups of students. Each semester that I have taught in this manner, the progression of the students remains the same (i.e., start with dislike, then move to a more active aggression, opposing it until the end when most find the course extremely valuable). I have tried to explain to the students that, course content aside, they were getting tremendous value in their work experience by contributing to this project – just by getting exposure with little or no risk. None of these assurances has been able to speed the students through the technology adoption curve. In fact, here it is much worse because the technology is wrapped up in the re-engineering of the course. Therefore, their aggressive ignorance is heightened by the fact that too many things are changing – the technology *and* the process (which we will come back to in a later section).

The role of the consumer

In the banking section, we described the change phenomenon around new technologies in two areas: the loan officer's decision and the customers' ATM usage and access to credit-risk rating information. In this education setting, we once again have two stakeholder groups: this time there are the faculty members giving the course and the students. The focus of my experience here is on the students and attempting to both implement new technology and then expedite their passage through the technology adoption curve. I limited the story to the student as a consumer as I felt that this would relate better to the later discussion of the patient as a consumer.

When I first entered the undergraduate Commerce and Administration program at Concordia University (in Montreal) over 25 years ago, we as students had very little information with which to make decisions. All of the information that we were provided was standard literature about the program, the school (which had just formed in 1974 from the merger of Loyola College and Sir George Williams

University) and very limited blurbs about courses in the calendar. I did not visit the school before making my decision and had no opportunity to compare one university to the next. Certainly, there was no information available on teacher evaluations or rankings on universities or colleges; in fact there was no measurement of any kind, regardless of how flawed it may have been.

At the time that notices were sent to the students confirming their acceptance into the university, we also received an invitation to come to the campus for pre-registration in order to select the courses for the first year. We were given a room number and a specific appointment time. In my case, I was scheduled to be there at 8:30 am one Wednesday morning in late August 1976. Unfortunately, I did not realize that everyone else entering the first year undergraduate business program was also given the same date, time and location. We then queued up in various lines for different courses for differing amounts of time. At one point I waited three hours only to be told that section of the course was now full and that the only option was 4:15pm Mondays and Wednesdays. In and of itself, that would not have been too bad. The problem was that I had already been forced into an 8:45 to 10:00 am for the only other course scheduled on Mondays and Wednesdays (which were required courses for the degree), leading to a very ineffective schedule.

Needless to say, by the end of the day, there were many frustrated students who all seemed to have various inefficiencies in their schedules for the first two semesters. Surely, there had to be a better way! Perhaps, by "incenting" frustration, the University found a very ingenious method of getting first year students to think about administration and the management of large organizations as they entered post-secondary education in business. Perhaps not!

Through many years of trial and error, the one major source of frustration and angst, course registration (especially in the first year), has improved, due in large part, to information technology. In today's university (as well as other levels of education), students can either dial in using interactive voice response (IVR) or log on through the Internet and peruse all types of data on course options. They can see course outlines online and even review the whole degree curricula, before making choices about courses they want or to which programs they would like to apply. When the students have made their choices, they can select and confirm their registration without ever having to go down to the campus. Within a matter of minutes, a once-painful exercise can be completed – with increased efficiency and effectiveness. Students can now knowledgeably select the schedule that is optimal for them (given certain constraints, of course). Moreover, many universities hold "course fairs" where students and faculty (and/or advisors) can interact to learn more about the course detail (workload and grading expectations) before they select their courses.

In addition to the process of course selection and registration, consumerism has had other dramatic effects in the education world. The branch of distance education has allowed those in even the remotest areas to avail themselves of a post-secondary education at the best of schools. Further, where once students had little choice as to what university to attend, they now have many options as well as many delivery choices (e.g., part-time, full-time executive, traditional on-campus). With the course detail and curriculum information on the Web, students do have options and universities now truly compete (even on national levels) for the best students. This competition is further enhanced by university rating initiatives that have been growing in popularity – perhaps the most well-known in Canada is the *Maclean's* magazine issue that comes out rating universities in a number of categories by a suite of different criteria each fall.

Although many argue that the criteria are either not fair, not reliable or not valid (usually presented by those universities that score below average), it's a beginning and more and more people are paying attention to the ratings when they start thinking of the best place for themselves or their children's education. In fact, many executives in universities have changed their focus from one of complaining about the rating to one of trying to influence the criteria in order to place the comparisons on a more equal footing – "If you can't beat them, join them!" Once again, better technology and better information has improved the decision-making process for the users of the system – and in this case, the students. We have come a long way by making information accessible and thereby creating competition and making the stakeholders more accountable.

4. Level of consumer (or end-user) influence during early stages of adoption

The influence of consumerism has also made it all the way into the classroom. Once the domain of the teacher, the classroom has now become much more of a meeting of minds on a more or less equal playing field. (I described above the need to be able to force students to employ DET; this is too strong a tone for this day and age – perhaps it's more a combination of forcing and lobbying!) Students are less intimidated by the faculty and are willing to challenge when they feel that expectations are unrealistic or if they disagree with the content. This has all led to a much more exciting place for debate and growth. In my undergraduate days, there was very little challenging as we listened to the sage on the stage so to speak. Now, we see the teacher as being more of a facilitator and the students are the ones often leading the discussions, especially in graduate school. Faculty members are now much more a guide on the side.

Before we leave this section, let's examine the healthcare industry in this context. I have stated that years ago the students had very little knowledge about what courses were being offered, about the degree program itself (and the institution for that matter) and about the level of expectation in the classroom in order to achieve a good result. Further, students had very little control over their schedule. Does this remind anyone of healthcare today? Let's see: we have very little knowledge about hospital performance, which doctors do what procedures and the types of potential outcomes, and the patient surely has no input into when they can see their physician!

Also, we have no comparisons regarding hospital performance in the way we now do with the universities. I agree that there is room for improvement in university rankings but, at least, it is a start.

Finally, how much influence does the consumer (patient) have when they do not agree with their doctor – can they influence the decisions that are made regarding their health? How many patients have exercised their options and selected a different hospital or doctor because of the service they have received – and more importantly, how many people felt comfortable about it. I believe we are still a long way from having effective competition in healthcare to the point where we have real delivery options. Therefore, we must create awareness, competition and measurement – and all of this can only be achieved through better system information.

Performance measurement

We can analyze the performance measurement topic from many angles. We can review the performance of the organization (i.e., a balanced scorecard, where the evaluation is across a number of indicators, or one individual dimension such as winning the Stanley Cup in professional hockey), specific individual performance measures themselves (reduction in loan losses for a bank's credit card portfolio) or the performance of the technology itself (in terms of efficiency or speed of analysis or with respect to overall user satisfaction in working with the system to obtain access to grades or course materials and handouts). In the end, did the technology assist the students in making better decisions? Are the students better off? Have they learned more?

Measuring students' overall knowledge is difficult enough let alone being able to compare it to a previous point in time. This would be akin to asking if shoppers are better consumers after purchasing a product off the Internet. In sports, perhaps we can use a quantitative measure (such as won-loss record) but how can you assign a measure as to whether the entire class of students actually learned the curriculum – and whether they learned more than last year's class that did not have the advantage of, say, new technology? (I will call it an "advantage" until it is proven otherwise.) Perhaps, one of the best ways is to just ask the students.

Have we improved the decision making of the students? I believe, for all of the reasons stated above, the answer must be yes. The main reason for success here is that there was a large investment in training at the outset of the semester(s) and a lot of support throughout the projects. This then allows the student to become very familiar and confident with the new technology to the point where they begin to focus on the problems they're facing and less on the technology component.

5. Level of effective reporting on the status of the outcome measures during and post implementation

Reporting is often thought of as printed results of data, information – perhaps measures or indicators. However, reporting can also take the form of verbal and visual feedback on the progress of the development and implementation of a system. In this educational setting, there was more control over the users than there may be in other settings where the usage has to be influenced or seduced. Therefore, reporting can be seen as a critical component of building momentum and an incentive for continued commitment to the project.

In a university course, students can be forced to use the new technology by assigning a grade component to their utilization and evaluation, which is precisely what we did. Over time, if the technology is not effective, resistance will result and will be much more organized, often in the form of complaints to the faculty member or to the administrative component of the curriculum – or even the Dean's office if need be. However, in the short term, a situation can be created where you force the users to ride through the early part of the adoption curve (over the top at Time 3) so that they begin to experience for themselves the benefits that arise at Time 4 and beyond. This component of this story is critical and must not be overlooked when comparing it to the upcoming hockey example.

6. Level of effectiveness in dealing with good or bad fortune

In this case study, we mentioned two different and distinct stakeholder groups: the students and the faculty members. Our focus to this point has been exclusively on the students. However, unlike the students, the faculty cannot be forced to do anything in their domain – which is primarily the delivery of their courses and the methodologies that they choose to implement. This would be considered infringement on academic freedom and the stifling of both the science and the art of education. As a result, the faculty were very slow in adopting the new technology. This led to mixed signals to the students who became very unsure as to the future of DET in the program.

It was at a very critical point in the adoption that we got lucky. The students began to put pressure on the faculty to make the change. The few early adopter faculty members had convinced the few early adopter students that the technology had merit. They then influenced the remaining student body who then sought out the remaining faculty's buy-in so as to ensure that there would be consistency across all the teachers in the program. As with the students, the faculty then needed to be trained, have technical support and have their own input into the features of the DET selected. Ultimately, it was pressure from the students that led (or perhaps forced) the faculty to adopt this new technology.

This reminds me of the story of three university professors who are walking down the beach and they stumble over a magic lamp. Knowing his history, one of them started to rub the lamp and a genie popped out. He was so elated to be freed that he granted them three wishes – one each, but a year between each one. The first professor said that he wanted to be the best teacher in the entire world. The genie thought for a second and then waved his hands in the air. A certain confidence fell over the first professor and over the next year, he began to excel in his field, giving talks and presentations all around the globe.

On the first anniversary of their meeting, the three professors returned to the same beach. As promised, the genie returned and asked the second professor what he wanted. Of course, he responded that he wanted to be the best teacher on earth (obviously these guys were a little competitive!). The genie thought a little longer and then waved his hand again. And, sure enough, over the next year, the second professor received even more notoriety than the first and gained tremendous prominence to the point that one could argue that he was now the best in the world.

On the second anniversary, all were assembled and the genie awaited the response from the third professor. You guessed it – he wanted to be the best teacher in the world. The genie then said that this would take some serious thought, as he wasn't sure how even he could out-do himself a second time. After a few minutes, he turned to the third professor and said that he would make him the best teacher in the world … and poof, he turned him into a student!

We must never stop learning and it is in this way that we can become the best teachers.

THE HOCKEY STORY

I had the opportunity a few years ago to spend some time with the Vancouver Canucks Hockey Club. I had worked with a couple of National Hockey League coaches on developing some software for game video and data analysis. I travelled with the team from mid-season through to the seventh game of the Stanley Cup Finals. There were many great experiences, but the one constant component that kept haunting the team was the lack of a sense of urgency. Over an eighty-four game schedule, it's tough to retain a sense of consistency – however, the good teams do it better than the poor ones. Maintaining a consistent level of importance in their play or urgency is imperative. Unless the players exhibit that level of play that can best be described as "will not lose" (which is different from "afraid to lose or to make a mistake"), that elite level of play is not attainable.

It seemed that our team only played that way when we really had to – when we were on the verge of elimination. That playoff season, we faced elimination 6 times and won five of those games. The record in the playoffs was 12 wins and two losses over one stretch – not bad for a team (against the league's best competition, mind you) that could not escape the five hundred winning percentage mark all season (i.e., fifty percent wins and fifty percent losses).

Creating change

I developed a software package, with assistance from many parties, called SHARP (Statistical Hockey Analysis and Reporting Package). In essence, this software allows for the development and management of a database of hockey information. This database management system (DBMS) plays two roles: it acts as a (1) database to organize all relevant data and information; and (2) it is a decision support system (DSS) that helps the hockey manager, at all levels, make decisions that can be fully supported with the necessary facts.

In hockey, much of the data on players' performance comes from on-going review of the game videotapes. In addition to the coaching staff employing these tapes for strategy formulation, this information can be used as a teaching tool where the player himself requires feedback. Historically, the recording of game-related data had all been done by hand and was stored in filing cabinets in the coaches' office. The game highlights were all stored on videotape and kept on shelves above the coaches' desks. As one can imagine, this leads to a very cumbersome, if not non-existent, retrieval system. If there was a query or search that needed to be addressed that required the data and video to be integrated, then the tasks became almost overwhelming.

The computer system that I created in 1994 – at a time in the early 1990s before digital video became commonplace – stored all of the data and video right on the computer hard disk. In this way, all of the information was fully integrated (because it was saved that way) and was available almost instantly. Thus, if a coach required, for example, to see the statistics on all scoring chances from the power play in the last five minutes of a game when the team is down by a goal against another team, the system can provide that information almost immediately. Further, if he wanted to see these particular chances in video form, the clips can be shown with the same degree of expediency right there on the computer screen. No filing cabinets, no VCR hookups, no TV. As long as the data and the video had been saved digitally, we could have the information sliced up and presented any way the coaches wanted it.

Once developed in the lab, the system needed to be tested. After all the years of preparation, research and system development, I went about trying to get someone, some team, to employ the system. I didn't care particularly where – just somewhere to see if it really did add value. If this proved to be the case, then other coaches and other teams would be more willing to use it. The New York Rangers and the Vancouver Canucks were both interested. So interested, in fact, that they were willing to lend me their teams, as it were, to give the system a serious test; the Rangers for a four-year period (1989–1993) to develop a prototype and the Canucks to test the system in a "live environment" (1993–94 season). The opportunity to test my system to the fullest was critical to its success.

I documented this progress over a five-year period, from creative idea to early prototypes to finished product to technology adoption to implementation.

Over the course of the first half of the 1989–90 season during prototype development, the Rangers regularly sent game tapes to me – usually a shipment once every two weeks and normally with six or seven videotapes at a time. The analysis was going so well that, during one of my conversations with Ron Smith, assistant coach of the Rangers at the time, I suggested that I meet the team during their west coast trip.

I had created a statistic called *scoring chances per minute played*. From this, Brian Mullen was at the top of the list. Mullen was routinely on the third or fourth line and did not play nearly as much as the club's top wingers. This "new" statistic now revealed that on a "per minute played" basis, he was contributing more than any other player on the team. (Of course, these two facts are not unrelated; it may be that as his ice and playing time increases, his performance declines due to lack of stamina, skills, etc. However, explanations notwithstanding, it was an interesting observation.) At the end of the meeting, I left the coaches with my analysis and reports. The outcome of the game? Well, the Rangers won by a score of 4–1. Brian Mullen scored two goals and assisted on one other. He was first star. Probably just a coincidence …

> *It should be noted here that a large reason for the successful implementation of the first version of this information system was the contribution of the team's assistant coach as an early adopter. This resulted in tremendous buy-in. There is a need for performance measurement; and if the right measurement does not exist, then new metrics must be created to communicate the innovation and improvement.*

During the following season's training camp, I spent more time with the coaching staff. It became obvious that some things that I had taken for granted were not true. First, not everyone likes computers. Perhaps, even more revealing was the fact that not everyone sees the computer as an asset – as a tool that can make life and jobs much easier. In fact, I was told by one assistant coach that he has "yet to see a computer ever score a goal" – a very difficult argument to refute! This resistance to change and to computers was going to provide difficulties.

Perhaps an outgrowth of the first observation was the fact that not everyone knows (or wants to know) how to type and use a computer. The system that I had developed did not require much in the way of straightforward typing but it did require a familiarity with a keyboard. This familiarity was non-existent. Further, lack of experience with computers meant that there would be problems with software installation in the case of up-grades and with day-to-day operations, just in terms of making back-up copies of the database.

The remainder of my time was spent training the coaches and making sure the system could do what the coaches wanted it to do. This meant reviewing the data that was to be captured and the format of the reports. Once we agreed on that, I determined what system modifications needed to be made to make the system not only user-friendly, but in the case of some individuals, user-seductive.

*As can be seen, I involved the coaching staff, through training and system design, so they could have as much input into the development of the system as possible. In this way, it was becoming less my system and more **our** system.*

As the long season was approaching the end, the Rangers were concerned about the system. The major limitation in 1991 was that the statistical package, no matter how thorough, was separate from the videotapes that contained all their game highlights. Statistics are fine, but how does one improve on these statistics? For example, the stats may prove that a certain player is weak on chances against on the rush. That's great information but what do you do with it?

The system must be used or it is not of any value. Do you no longer play that player – bench him, trade him? Or do you try to get that player to improve? The best solution is the latter, of course. And the best way to improve a situation is to examine the way things are currently being done – hence the need to go back to the game tapes. Therefore, if the Rangers, or any other team, were going to be interested in this new information system, there must be a link between the video and the statistics. Otherwise, what I had was neat, but there was no competitive advantage over other systems.

Clearly, my next step was to examine state-of-the-art multi-media capabilities and learn to apply those capabilities to the world of sport. At times, system development ideas often exceed the current capabilities of technology – this is not unique to sports. However, one positive is when the idea for innovation emanates from the user or client, then they are usually willing to implement eventually (at least on a test basis) due to the fact that they were part of the design process – quite independent of the period of time that we all spent waiting for technology to catch up.

By the fall of 1993, I had created a prototype; as with applications in any industry, no one really knows the true impact of innovation until they see it operational. This was my biggest challenge, to show an NHL team management (now the Vancouver Canucks) that a fully integrated information system can not only be of value, but can also be the integral processing unit for sports decision-making.

One of the major ways that I was able to get my information system "accepted" was by presenting the reports in exactly the same layout as the previous versions that were hand-written. So, I used a special hand-written-like font from the Mac and left reports on the coaches' desks immediately after games. Some of the coaches started to wonder who had done their reports so fast. Up until this point, some of the coaches never even looked at my information; with the right layout and font, the reports were getting more recognition, at least initially, for the speed of turnaround than for their additional and innovative content. Not great, but it got the coaches started in the right direction.

Toward the end of the regular season, change could be observed in the coaches' behaviour. Although, I do not believe that a single computer programmer or computer system can make that big a difference, it can play a large role. First of all, someone new close to the top of management can often be seen as a catalyst. This brings new optimism and energy. This alone can bring a team some focus and determination. Second, the computer video system has freed up the coaches to spend less time with their VCRs and more time doing what they should be doing, coaching the players. I believe this is the biggest contribution – the computer system enables coaches to afford the time to use information in their jobs rather than the other way around – using their time trying to find the information.

In the playoffs, the intensity of the coaches' preparation began escalating. Further, for some reason, the coaches started going back and resorting to their old ways of doing things! One exception was our goalie coach who was interested in watching all our goals for in games against Calgary (our first round opponent) in the regular season. I was able to bring them right to the computer screen, sorted by game, almost instantly. Deep down, I was very proud of that accomplishment.

From then on however, even though I continued to offer my services, I was consulted very little. We went on to win three rounds and lost the Cup in game seven of the finals by one goal!

At this point, it may have become evident that I was not considered to be an essential cog in the decision-making process for the team. It's important to remember that I was brought on to pilot a new information system. Over the first couple of playoff series, after we had proven that the computer system was effective, the research was considered complete. Since then, the system had just been running in the background, doing the odd statistical report. The video component had not yet been incorporated into the coaching preparation – waiting until next season (and a new coach?) before going to full implementation. Why weren't they using the system to its fullest extent? The pilot study had proven to be successful – we were in the Finals – Game Seven! Just from a superstition perspective, you'd think they'd want to keep using it. Plus the main advantage, in addition to better information, was that it allowed the coaches to coach and not be "paper-jockeys."

To end on a more positive note, the new technology was implemented into the NHL and an investment of time and money was made. This was only accomplished after four years of hard work and a one-year trial adoption period. I stated earlier that the objective of achieving a more patient-focused health system could take about ten years – and that may be an optimistic view. However, as of the 2003–2004 hockey season, a large percentage of hockey teams now employ some variant of the system we piloted in 1993–94. Ultimately, the adoption took many years, but it did eventually take place and would never have happened if not for our early work.

Takeaways from the story

- So, what can we learn from this story? Why did the system have so little effect – especially in the last round of the playoffs, which, one could argue, was the most important time for an effective information system?

    These are a couple of the major questions that have haunted me for some time following the end of that season. I think there are a number of answers.

First, as a system developer, I was very much in awe of the hockey industry and the key people in it. Instead of going about the business of designing a decision support system for coaches, at times I lost my perspective and respected the industry too much. It was an industry that had worked well without me and as such, what value could I add? If system developers are to be change agents, then we must not be intimidated by the industry players and not be afraid to make change! In the end, I needed to be more of an advocate for the new system and less of a fan of the Vancouver Canucks and the management that ran the team.

Second, there was tremendous, and well organized, resistance to change. A couple of key players in team management were constantly lobbying against the system. Instead of addressing this head-on, I retreated to a safer position and was content to call this a research project or pilot study. The fact is that this was a chance to make change in an industry that has been slow to adopt new technology and I should have addressed the change issue much more directly. Since I did not, I was constantly undermined, constantly on the run. A large part of the resistance is from the amount of work that it takes to learn a new system – and to basically run two systems at the same time. Ron Smith invested four years to learn the system but others were not as eager to be involved in this technology and therefore, we never got to the point where the workload started to decrease (i.e., the ever elusive Time 4 on Figure 1, page 27).

After much reflection, I have arrived at six conditions that define winning the Stanley Cup, the trophy defining supremacy in the NHL. These are:

- Quality and skill level of players – with draft, computers and information services and with free agency there is pretty much a level playing field
- Coaching systems – many different – that get players on the same page – no one system is better than any other but they need a system
- Level of commitment of each and every player
- Ability of each player to flourish within the coach's system
- Reporting or providing feedback on the performance to date
- Handling the good or bad lucks, the breaks.

Simply, you must have the talent, a good coaching plan, a way to get the most out of the players, have the players excel, keep providing feedback and effectively handle both good and bad luck! As one can see, the six hockey conditions are the exact same as the CSFs outlined throughout this book. Let's examine the first three here.

1. Amount of industry experience in using technology

This industry has virtually no experience and as such, would require a very long period between Times 1 and 3 on the technology adoption curve. Some of this movement can be managed or expedited but much will just move at its own pace and that must be recognized.

2. Amount of training both before and during the transition

Other than Ron Smith, a very keen early adopter, there was very little training done on the system and very little background given on why we were doing it. Looking back, an overall introduction presentation should have been done when I joined the team; in fairness we did that, but not everyone attended.

3. Amount of buy-in (or contribution during design) from the different stakeholder groups

Other than a couple of key people over the first five years, we did not involve other stakeholders as the system development progressed. In retrospect, we needed to have these design/development meetings every month so that others could have had their input and we could have potentially earned their buy-in.

The role of the consumer

At first glance, it may appear that consumerism has had very little effect on the game of hockey. Unlike the music industry, for example, it's not entirely obvious how the "will of the average consumer" has had an effect on the direction of the industry. In music, there has been a tremendous rise in awareness of the state of the industry and a desire to get music as soon as it is released and for the lowest possible cost. One great example is the Napster debate and the need for legislation to halt the widespread, and unauthorized, distribution of new releases without royalties (or commission) going to the creative artist. Here, the public demand created a whole new industry that spawned MP3 players and so on and this effect is clearly evident.

Returning to hockey, it may be difficult to see what has changed and how the consumer actually played a critical role in that change. To see this, however, we must go back a few decades. In the 1960s (when I was first watching hockey on television as a child), we would get only one game a week on TV – Saturday night and Hockey Night in Canada (HNIC) on CBC Television. Occasionally a mid-week game was televised (usually a Wednesday night) but this was infrequent and anything but predictable. Because televised games were still in their infancy (regular radio broadcasts started in the 1930s and HNIC began in 1952), there was still a fear that broadcasting the game on TV would hurt live attendance and gate receipts (in many ways this is still prevalent today in the Canadian Football League, or CFL, with home games being blacked out on occasion).

In order to ensure that the attendance was at its maximum possible, the broadcast of the games on CBC Saturday night used to start one-half hour after the game started. The games were not broadcast in full on a tape delay (there was no such thing back then) but rather televised live, missing the first 30 minutes of action – normally accounting for a large percentage of the first period (unless there had been an injury or a fight). In fact, at many parties and Saturday night get-togethers, one of the hot topics of conversation centred on trying to guess the score of the game before it started. (A common joke was always guessing zero-zero, but the intention was to guess the score at the start of the broadcast and not the actual start of the game!)

Now, fast forward to the 2003–2004 hockey season where every single game of the 82-game season for all 30 teams is now broadcast somewhere – and in its entirety, I might add. Overall attendance figures, advertising revenue and, ultimately, television viewership now indicate that there is a demand for this product. In the world of big business and economics, the name of the game is supply and demand. If the demand is there, then one had better have the supply or someone else will deliver it.

Forty years ago, CBC was the only network broadcasting hockey games nationally anywhere. In fact, for many years, there was simply no demand in the United States to televise hockey other than regionally for specific markets. However, with growing interest in the sport, ABC and ESPN both began broadcasting hockey nationally in the US. And if they didn't then someone else would. In Canada, TSN now has the national rights to games not televised by CBC. (In fact, television networks pay hundreds of millions of dollars for the rights to broadcast team games, monies which have eventually gone to both the owners and the players in these sports –

thereby inflating salaries and unfortunately, ticket prices.)

Further, on Saturday nights, for the last number of years, HNIC has covered two games – an Eastern Time zone game starting at 7pm EST (following a half hour of pre-game hype) and a late game usually originating in Alberta or Vancouver. Can you imagine what the response from the public would be if CBC stopped covering the Leafs' games on Saturday night, if they missed a playoff game or even if they just started the broadcast one-half hour into the game? And you thought there was no consumerism in hockey!

The consumerism doesn't stop there. The viewing public has also shut down new ideas such as the glowing puck that The Fox Network originated a few years ago. It was their idea that the audience would follow the play better if the puck glowed when it moved. It was not a huge success and the fans/consumers provided that feedback.

Not all ideas are perfect, but the attempt to improve the technology related to the broadcast should be applauded and recognized. In fact, it's my opinion that we should all fail at our jobs somewhere between 5 to 10 percent of the time, especially in the system design field. If we don't then we're not trying to reach beyond our grasp, we're not challenging ourselves enough and as a result, we're not learning because we're not pushing the creative bounds to the point where we fail from time to time. Further, I believe that performance evaluation must also include a component measuring how much one fails: whether it's too much or too little – and both must be discouraged. Too much failure may hurt the bottom line; but not enough risk will surely kill a company's creative advantage in the long term.

Another large effect on hockey, and sports in general, is the insatiable appetite that consumers have for devouring the statistics on their favourite teams and players. Years ago, the only statistics one would see in the newspaper the day following a game were the team standings (recording wins, losses, ties, points and so on) and the players' own totals regarding goals and statistics. Over time, these have evolved to include time on ice, scoring chances, shots, scoring percentage (as a percentage of shots) and plus-minus stats. These are now recorded and published because there is a demand to see them. Further, new technology has facilitated the generation of these statistics (i.e., computers), but the ultimate demand originates with the consumer.

4. Level of consumer (or end-user) influence during early stages of adoption

In the end, the consumer has had much effect on the direction of hockey (as well as other forms of entertainment), eventually increasing the market opportunity for suppliers. This is the key point: The suppliers have not been threatened by the rise in consumerism but rather see this as a tremendous opportunity to capitalize on the demand for products and services. If anything, suppliers of entertainment have tried to fan the flame of consumer interest as opposed to dousing it with negative attitudes and rhetoric. In the end, they have created a market for information whereby the information, segmented into standard packages, becomes a marketable product. One good example of this is the creation of new sports channels dedicated to one specific team – the Maple Leaf Channel and the Yankees Entertainment and Sports (YES) network to name but two.

Performance measurement

Did the information system provide value-add to the team? Following Game Six of the Finals, the head coach and general manager and I sat down and talked for a few minutes about the year behind us and the one game that was ahead. We talked about personal gains and losses and the lessons learned. It's difficult for me, even now, to fully comprehend the accomplishment that we achieved. It is only over time that we will truly appreciate the significance of our work during that year. Yet, even though we accomplished much, much more than anybody thought we would, the ending was filled with disappointment. Many people that I have talked to have tried to convince me that the team had a great year – and we did. But when you are this close to the ultimate, there can be no solace in getting close; you must grab victory.

Heading into the playoffs in mid-April, all we wanted to do was play well, represent our fans and do the franchise justice. As the series progressed, we went from wanting to win the next game to wanting to win it all. Somewhere during the Finals, we began to expect the best from ourselves and to demand the best outcome. In a way, that was the precise moment when we became true winners – when we got to know ourselves, and to respect ourselves and our work. Although it's disappointing not to win the championship (something that will live on forever), we did find the desire within ourselves to achieve the best – and that's also something that no one will ever be able to take away from us! This, I believe, is the component of character that teams are looking for in the leaders that have won championships in the past.

The haunting question, however, still remains: Did we do a good job – or, in other words, was the one-year consulting task for this NHL team successful? How do we measure this success? What is the real outcome measure? Is it winning the Stanley Cup? Is it taking the team farther into the playoffs than it had ever been before? Did the information system make a difference? Would the team have gone that far without it? Would it – could it have gone farther? (Of course, any farther than the third period of game seven, by definition, means winning the Stanley Cup.)

The answers to many of these questions present this project, and ultimately the information system, in a very positive light. The team did go farther than the previous year; indeed, the Vancouver franchise had never gone further in its history (since 1970) than we did this year. (Although it is true that the Canucks made the Finals in 1982, they were eliminated by the New York Islanders in four straight games.)

I guess the question of the highest import is: Did we advance the use of, and the appreciation for, new technology in the world of professional sport (i.e., hockey)? To be truthful, the answer must be yes and no. In the short term, did the Canucks continue using the information system the subsequent year? The answer is no. At the most critical time, game seven, did the management employ the system that they invested a whole season to develop in order to take competitive advantage in the most important area – information? No, I was not even considered significant enough to warrant flying on the same plane with the coaches back to New York for game seven. In fact, I was not even in the arena when we were eliminated. By any true measure, this was a personally satisfying year; however, professionally, it was more a disappointment than a successful software experiment and implementation.

To provide a fair evaluation, however, we must look farther down the road. We did state that the point of the exercise the first season was to pilot the system and have a full implementation and evaluation during the subsequent season. And, although there are many reasons for a team's success, I believe the software contributed to some degree by making the coaches more productive. This success notwithstanding, the following season started with a players' strike and owners' lockout (collapsing it to 48 games starting in January of 1995) and then a new head coach was selected. Unfortunately, my future with the Canucks became tenuous and the software became the first casualty of restructuring.

On the other hand, even though we never did get to the full implementation (i.e., never beyond the prototype stage), systems design work is very important at whatever stage it's in – and the evaluation of it takes place whether we are ready or not. Perhaps, the most important lesson of all is that we are all being constantly evaluated and so we must always do the best we can do – at work or in life. As of the beginning of the 2003–2004 hockey season, many teams have now successfully adopted similar coaching IS to what we first pioneered. From this perspective, I believe that we were very successful.

At the end of my last teaching semester (April 2004), I had a student approach me and say: "Professor Leonard, if I had one hour left to live I would want to live it in your class." Well, to say that I was taken aback would be an understatement! Not being one to leave well enough alone, I proceeded to ask a follow-up question. Why? Was it my wit, command of the subject matter, fair evaluation? "No," she responded, "nothing like that – it's that an hour in your class goes on forever." See, whether we like it or not, we're constantly being evaluated!

5. Level of effective reporting on the status of the outcome measures during and post implementation

If we had established objective outcomes measures at the beginning of the project, we could have monitored these measures through time and gained momentum, enthusiasm and more widespread acceptance. In addition and in fairness, the timing of the system development was such that video quality was at a point where computer video was a bit choppy in quality, which hurt the prestige of the project; so much so that the industry was simply not at a point where there were enough early adopters to keep a project such as this alive through the next iteration and implementation.

What is the relationship between the technology investment and the performance measure – and is it required? It's extremely difficult just to answer this question let alone provide all of the statistical evidence because there are many factors that impact the particular outcome being measured. Ideally we would have a randomized trial or parallel universes but this wasn't feasible for obvious reasons. Producing measures as the project progresses is definitely one way to illustrate the development and stakeholders are more likely to accept the final results if they have been part of the process through time. That was my biggest oversight in this industry and ultimately led to a longer technology adoption cycle.

6. Level of effectiveness in dealing with good or bad fortune

In an industry that recognizes the good bounce phenomenon more than most, it's ironic that here was one case where I did not take advantage of this issue. We never truly discussed the measurement of the system. We never defined a specific outcome in order to determine, objectively, whether or not the project met its goals. Only an inexperienced consultant would take on a task and not know how he/she was going to be measured. (I guess I qualify!) The team subsequently ran a streak of good fortune and with the right measures early on, we could have proven a strong relationship between better information and improved outcomes – if for no other reason than just good timing. Unfortunately, I didn't take advantage of this good fortune!

CONCLUDING COMMENTS
FROM THE THREE STORIES

Let's revisit the issue of the technology assisting its own adoption. The challenge in the banking story was to provide evidence that technology would work for a specific portfolio, and if so, provide an estimate of the profits or savings or both. Credit scoring has brought with it new technology needed to calculate and manage the scores. Computer systems have been developed that allow different types of strategy to run in parallel with completely different sets of rules and policies. In order to mimic a research-style environment, the individual assignment of any one account to a specific strategy is done on a completely random basis – removing any type of potential for system or personnel bias (using an RCT – a randomized "credit" trial, if you will).

Therefore, the adoption of new technology in credit has moved away from a theoretical argument to a more practical question of implementing various strategies and technology on small percentages of the portfolio. The results then indicate the next steps and the guesswork is removed from the adoption. For example, if the test does not add value then all that we have done is tried something creative and it failed to improve the performance; this is not a bad accomplishment given any organization's need to grow and learn in order to survive. If it does add value, then the facts provide the hard results that make the case for a larger percentage of the port-folio to be rolled out in order to take full advantage of the new technology.

Would it not be great if we could do that same type of testing in all of the industries that we have discussed so far in this book? How about hockey teams playing two different series – such as the Canucks and the Flames in the first round of the 1994 playoffs? We could play one against the Flames with information and then one without it and see the dif-ference! Or maybe we could have played some of the individual games in the series with the new technology and some without it. This is simply not possible but even if we did try it, how would we hold everything else constant – for example, player performance, travel, injuries, refereeing? If we couldn't, then the resistors to change could always credit the improvement to a variation in the other conditions and not the new tech-nology. I guess there are always a million reasons not to do something – and only one to actually do it – and that's the only way we learn.

Carrying the analogy one step further, what if we let some of the students have access to the Web material and some not, and then evaluate how each group performs on midterm exams or assignments? Once again, I'm not sure how feasible this would be. But the message is important; with the right performance measures, the move through the technology adoption curve is expedited.

Finally, in healthcare, we have a history of "live testing" called RCTs or randomized clinical trials. These trials do this exact same thing – for instance, a double blind scenario has some of the patients getting a new drug and others not; both the patients and the clinicians are unaware as to which patients receive which treatment. So if there is any industry that is prepared to utilize this philosophy it would be healthcare. However, to date, we have not constructed this type of environment for testing newer systems and better information (except for some rare and exceptional cases).

The single hurdle most responsible for the delay is the lack of an accepted form of performance measurement and standards of calculation. In banking, we have loan losses, but we have nothing in healthcare to date that is uniformly accepted as a measure of health outcomes or technology contribution – we must work toward this type of performance measure.

"The lesson to learn from the experience is: the tougher the resistance to change, the more a joint effort of all affected groups that represent patients' interest is required. What counts is the shared effort and energy, and what has the most impact is a strong uniform voice of patients."

The Patients Network,
Summer 1998, Volume 3, Number 2, page 12.

CHAPTER SIX

My healthcare story

This chapter pertains to my own health experiences from birth until today. My experience with healthcare and healthcare systems has been exhaustive. That's not to imply that I'm a dissatisfied consumer who's trying to write a book to get even – quite the contrary. I believe that I am a healthy forty-something today due mainly to the effectiveness and advancements within the Canadian and US healthcare systems. In addition, my experience with healthcare is not limited to myself. I have parents, grandparents and other relatives, like all of us, who, from time to time, have needed the attention of the medical profession. By and large, my overall experience has been very positive. However, as in many other industries, it could stand some improvements.

When this book was only in manuscript form, many reviewers provided feedback suggesting that this chapter be moved forward – perhaps to Chapter One or Two – because of the powerful motivation it provides. The reader would then be able to identify with this author, thus making the rest of the book more engaging. I refused that suggestion because I didn't want to make the book solely about me as a patient. I wanted the book to represent ideas for change because they are needed, not because I'm sick. In the end, I wanted to portray myself as a contributor and not as someone who does not contribute.

It may be difficult for someone who doesn't have a chronic illness to understand, but I didn't want to come across as a victim, but rather as a survivor (which is common for most chronically ill patients). Most importantly, it was essential that my suggestions be heard on their merit before understanding their origins.

Throughout this chapter, I examine the medical profession from a long-overlooked perspective, through the eyes of the patient. I make suggestions regarding changes that must occur if the efficiency within healthcare is to improve. Most importantly, I discuss the type of changes that must be made to improve the overall relationship between healthcare and its patients.

Due to the growing strain on the system, patients are going to have to become more and more responsible for their own health issues and problems – both in long-term maintenance and with episodic care. Patients are going to need to take charge when it comes to proper diagnosis, alternatives of treatment and short- and long-term recovery. Certainly, the system will be there for support, however, in the future – in the not too distant future – patients are going to have to be the driving force in managing their healthcare. I know this requires a change in thinking, and although I have discussed resistance to change at length, this fact must be recognized and accepted: *the patient is ultimately responsible for his or her own care!*

The only way to accomplish this is to virtually turn the current healthcare processes inside out. At present, the patients are the last ones with the information. If you don't believe this, just ask your doctor to explain the latest treatments to whichever diagnosis you prefer. If they have the time to explain it, they'll probably explain it to you in a language and with terms that will be incomprehensible to most lay people. This is because, traditionally, the information has been tailored to be delivered to medical professionals – people who have some eight years of graduate school training in specific medical fields. The information was never intended to be given out to patients, at least not directly. Therefore, in an age of right to information and Health Management Organizations (HMOs), even if patients wanted the relevant facts, there is no easy way to access them because they're not in any consistently understandable format.

As a result, many of the changes I recommend throughout this book are directed at improvements in Information Systems (IS) within healthcare. Because the field of information systems is complex, with topics ranging from issues of data capture (data entry) to report generation, we'll need to focus on many areas of healthcare delivery. The most important element, however, remains IS for patients. This implies that requirements must be satisfied throughout healthcare in order to provide for these changes in IS for patients. In other words, doctors, hospitals and pharmacists need to create information that is understandable to the general population. In that way, when patients request information, it will be available and accessible for general consumption.

One objective of this book is to educate patients as to the type of changes that need to be made throughout the industry and for patients, as a group, to demand them together. In this way, we get the information we need and healthcare gets the information support that is required to improve efficiency and effectiveness.

The prerequisite, of course, is to design and develop information systems for patients. Many people have asked research questions pertaining to patient satisfaction and quality, but gaining information for the patients' own use is an area that has not often been addressed. In the pages that follow, this will be our focus.

Creating change

I was introduced to the field of healthcare at an early age. I'm not referring here to childbirth – which would put most of us in the same category – but rather to the onset of allergy-induced, childhood asthma at age two. I spent numerous hours in doctors' waiting rooms and clinics, to the point where the mere sniff of rubbing alcohol can still give me shivers. For a child (and for an adult, for that matter), sitting in a doctor's office can be very traumatic. Therefore, every time I had a medical encounter, I would try to distract myself by thinking of ways to run the operation (no pun intended) more efficiently. I would examine the ways that the people in the office communicated with each other, the times that people arrived, and how long it took them to leave. This turned out to be great preparation for a career as an academic, researcher and consultant. I found that, almost without exception, I would spend quadruple, and sometimes quintuple, the time in the waiting room compared to the actual time spent with the doctor. I'm convinced that the word patient comes from the patience that is needed to sit in these waiting rooms.

I managed to survive childhood asthma (obviously), as well as a myriad of other health-related problems, to receive a doctorate in business administration. My field, not surprisingly, is statistics and information systems.

Over the last few years, I have become completely fasci-
nated by the healthcare industry. With funding cutbacks, the
time to actually implement some of my childhood efficiency-
producing ideas has finally arrived. The need for change –
significant change – is upon us. As a result, this is a great time
to be involved with research in healthcare.

I am a firm believer in the existing medical system as it
stands today. I am an experienced consumer of this system, and
am qualified to speak about the *user's* perspective. In addition,
I have been active as a researcher and, from this perspective as
well, I believe that improving efficiency is the only answer to
retaining the healthcare system, as we know it. This is not to
say that I do not believe in change in the structure of the
system itself because I do, very strongly.

I believe that we need integrated healthcare delivery
systems and community health information networks.
However, the backbone of each of these organizations and networks is improved information systems. It is the intent of this
book to explore healthcare information systems for all the different stakeholders. For example, it's easy to think about how
our family physician should and could operate more efficiently.
The same can be said as well for the departments and programs within hospitals. How much more effective could they
be if their information systems were improved? It does not,
and should not, end there. There should also be improved
communication of information between healthcare providers
and the different levels of government, between healthcare
providers and the community, and between the healthcare
providers themselves.

We must also demand improved information systems for
patients. We, the patients, are a significant stakeholder group,

but we are provided very little information. Even though it is the law, it's very difficult to get access to our own medical record – in full and, information concerning performance of hospitals (for example) regarding financial position or mortality rates is impossible to ascertain. A full listing of physicians and their areas of specialty and corresponding performance in each area is the type of information that we can only dream about. This is not to infer that "Big Brother" will not let us see them – but rather that this type of information does not exist, anywhere. You may argue that your medical chart exists – and this is correct, to some extent. However, a full comprehensive medical record that integrates information from all healthcare providers (covering the period from birth to present) still does not exist anywhere in Canada or in the United States in 2004.

In this chapter, I provide a brief of my medical history. If I am to encourage patients to stand up and be heard, then I must be willing to be first. Further, this will provide not only a framework for my comments and analysis in the subsequent chapters but also will supply some insight into the level and the different areas within healthcare that I have experienced. The chapters that follow will explore areas of my research and the opportunities we have as members in a community (both the US and the Canadian communities) to work together to save something that we have worked long and hard to develop and of which we are all very proud.

In a recent discussion during a University of Toronto MIS (management information systems) class in the Masters of Science program for Health Administration (MHSc), a question was posed to the class: Who is responsible for healthcare in our country? The answers varied: the doctors, the nurses, the administrators. Some even naïvely suggested the academics! Others insisted that government must save healthcare – pointing the finger at the parliaments across the country.

I believe that none of these answers is fully correct. All of these players have a significant contribution to make, however, ultimately, it is us, you and I, that must take responsibility for our own healthcare. We can no longer use the excuse that "no one told me smoking was dangerous!" We must, individually and collectively, educate ourselves about our health options and demand to be educated when the information is not forth-coming. Together we have a strong voice, but it is silent (and overlooked) if we do not speak up. Hopefully, this book will help motivate everyone to get involved in improving our own health and in saving our healthcare system. *This is the most important initiative that you will be involved within your lifetime after all, it's about saving your life's time!*

THE BEGINNINGS OF MY ELECTRONIC PATIENT RECORD (EPR)

One never quite forgets their first experience with anesthesia … no matter how hard they try.

There is nothing worse than the helplessness you feel when you awake from surgery and you try to remember who you are, but cannot. When you try to respond verbally or move a muscle, but cannot. When you feel like you should be in control but are not! It doesn't last that long – but long enough to be memorable. Anyone who has gone through general surgery has experienced this, this helplessness. It doesn't matter how many times you've experienced surgery, the post-operative feelings are the same.

For most people, this phenomenon occurs when you are just about to regain consciousness following surgery. That state when you're not sure whether you're still awake from before the surgery or whether the surgery has, in fact, just been completed. You hear someone calling a name – almost incessantly – yet you don't have the ability to answer. It's the moment just before you realize it's your name they're calling. It's that instant when none of the pieces fit together. For me, that lack of control is terrifying, and perhaps the worst thing about surgery.

Seconds, perhaps even only an instant, later you begin to regain control of your faculties. You begin to piece together all of the recent events that led to the surgery, often regrettably. I say regrettably because this helplessness is often followed immediately by the awareness of sharp pain (from one or many places), and by the realization that visitation from the relatives is imminent. I am not quite sure which of these two events leads to the most stress, the pain or the relatives.

When we reflect on healthcare, it's only natural to relate back to our own experiences within the industry. Someone who has had as much experience as I have is at least somewhat qualified to comment on the change (I hesitate to use the term "growth") in quality of care over the years. Unlike with other industries, we are all, in one way or another, current and/or eventual customers of healthcare. As a result, we are all qualified to comment on healthcare services. I would like to share some of the highlights of my healthcare experiences.

Perhaps my single, most vivid experience within healthcare is the post-operative haze. It's so ironic that this haze or help-lessness is such an appropriate metaphor for the current healthcare industry in Canada and the US. In some ways, we are just now recovering from massive surgery on the services offered over the last decade or so. Further, we have not progressed enough to know how well the surgery went nor, to some degree, even whether the patient (i.e., the healthcare system) can survive. However, continuing with this analogy, long-term success (and survival) is predicated on good post-operative practices. If the patient begins to put the right controls and measures in place, there is no reason not to believe that he or she can still lead a long, healthy and productive life.

January 24, 1960 – *Montreal, Quebec*

I was born in 1957 to a family in Montreal, the second of two boys. In early 1960, my brother was almost six years old while I was only two and a half. Like most middle class families at the time, my parents did the best they could to make ends meet. My father worked for Canadian National Railways in Purchasing. My mother was a stay-at-home, suburban wife. They had just purchased a new home with a *large* mortgage (with payments totaling $73 per month!). Food and clothing purchases were very carefully budgeted. There was very little room for unexpected expenses or luxuries. Even though healthcare can hardly be classified as a luxury, in 1960 most families very seldom included hospital expenses in their financial plan. (The Canada Health Act was passed only in 1966 and then updated in 1984.) In those days, if large hospital bills arose, a bank loan or second mortgage would have to be secured if family savings were not sufficient or available.

I was raised in a Roman Catholic home and, as a result, fish was cooked every Friday. Unfortunately, I was also born with an allergy to fish. My allergy is so severe that just the smell of the oils from the fish cooking can cause an allergic reaction – even anaphylaxis. (Anaphylaxis is an extremely severe allergic reaction that occurs very quickly, often within seconds, and can send the patient into shock and sometimes results in death.) Therefore, shortly before supper every Friday, I would go into an allergy-induced asthma attack. My parents had very little experience with illness, let alone asthma, and were, as a result, very unsure what to attribute my shortness of breath and difficulty with breathing to – other than a strict aversion to the weekend.

> *Due to ignorance and the potential large medical bill, at the time, it was not uncommon for most people to delay medical treatment. I don't mean to imply that my parents (or other parents of the day) were delinquent in their parenting duties, but rather financial situations and costs were factored into the decision-making process. This meant that instead of seeking treatment before an emergency or practising preventative medicine, parents waited until the last minute – to the point where they could not put off the decision any longer.*

One Friday in January, our last minute arrived – and I was taken to an emergency department during an asthma attack that appeared to be more serious than normal. Because there was no previous diagnosis, a number of precautions (and tests) were taken (at a cost) and I stayed in the hospital for a number of days before my breathing fully stabilized and the cause was finally determined. On my release, my parents were told that I had a fish allergy. As a result, I should not be fed fish!

Unfortunately, that was all they were told. They were *not* told to stop cooking fish. They were *not* told that the mere smell of fish had set off the asthma attack in the first place. It was then left solely up to me (and to my parents) to make sure that I stayed away from my allergens for the rest of my life.

Basically, there was very little, if any, education. My parents were given no guidance as to how to modify my diet or how to avoid fish by-products. Further, there seemed to be very little cause for concern for my long-term well-being. Of course, as we have learned over the years, allergies can be very serious and are often life threatening. It's imperative that all allergens be avoided. Further, the proper medication should always be accessible – and in the proper form. For people with anaphylaxis, the proper medication form is a syringe prepared with the correct dosage of epinephrine (called an EpiPen). If the onset of the reaction can take only seconds, then medication in pill form will not be effective.

In 1960, medical treatment was basically episodic treatment. We treated an illness or an emergency. Overall health promotion was virtually non-existent. Since we paid for healthcare on a case-by-case basis, it seems we got what we paid for.

July 28, 1971 – *Montreal, Quebec*

In grade 6 (age 12), I was one of the bigger kids in my class – well over 100 pounds and very active in sports. By the time I turned fourteen, I was still the same – literally. I was the exact same height and my weight was now measuring a meager 67 pounds. (I was the one that the 99-pound weaklings looked for to take out their frustrations.) From age 12 to 14, considerable growth should have taken place. However, I seemed to be regressing as opposed to progressing. *Why did this happen?* That was the question that occupied my parents' every waking hour.

In the fall of 1969, at age twelve, I began losing weight. The primary symptoms were severe pain and cramps. There was some vomiting, but those episodes were few. Basically, I was suffering from severe stomach cramps and a significant loss in appetite. Other than that there were no symptoms.

Oddly enough, I felt, to some degree, that the illness was my fault. Consequently, I kept the painful, cramping episodes secret. Even today, I'm still not quite sure why I kept the pain and disease a secret for a few months; maybe I realized that, subconsciously, the disease was very serious. (I have since learned that this is not uncommon, especially with symptoms and diseases that are nebulous and difficult to describe.) Unlike a broken leg where no one is at fault and the diagnosis is clear-cut, the symptoms and the illness were very mysterious. For this reason, I believe, I put off telling my parents that occasionally suffered from severe pain that was significant enough to make me stop whatever I was doing. Further, I could not accurately describe the pain, the cause of it or any way to make it better.

It didn't take long for my mind to link eating with pain and discomfort. Soon the desire for food – and consequently, the appetite – not only decreased but died in total. Significant weight loss was not far behind. As the weight loss and lack of appetite increased, my overall physical well-being deteriorated. My ability to fight my illness decreased further and I began progressing down a vicious health spiral.

One afternoon, at home just after school, my mother passed by my room and saw me writhing in pain on my bed clutching my stomach for support. Like all mothers, she was able to coax the truth out of me. When it was determined that I had been suffering from these pains for a few months, she began to seek help immediately.

Describing the pain and the symptoms, as it turned out, was not only my problem, but a problem that was shared by many. It seems that having stomach pains, loss of appetite and the occasional bout of vomiting were, for some reason, not enough information to pinpoint an accurate diagnosis. Therefore, after consulting our general practitioner (GP), we then saw the specialists. Unfortunately, most left us with the impression that we needed more tests – some physical and some not.

Because I was a middle child (a younger sister was born in 1961), when my parents began seeking medical help, the most popular preliminary diagnosis was that "he" was suffering from something called "middle child syndrome." (As an aside, I find it funny how often healthcare professionals refer to children in the third person – even when they're in the room – as opposed to including the child in the discussion – perhaps another book topic!) Being the second of three children in a family has distinct disadvantages, i.e., hand-me-down clothes, not being able to hang onto the friendly moniker of baby of the family – but I didn't know it automatically resulted in pain, cramping and vomiting. I began to worry about all the other families that I knew that had three children (and even ones I did not) and wondered whether the middle child was suffering physically as I was. I immediately thought that a law should be passed forcing parents to have either two or four children – but to never stop at three.

My parents explained that this syndrome was more of a mental condition than a physical one necessarily triggered when the parents decreed that they would stop the reproduction process at three siblings. I wondered then why the pain was physical and not mental! Upon reflection, it appeared that the mental component of this middle child syndrome was the worry that was brought on solely by being diagnosed as a potential "candidate."

During this "middle child syndrome diagnosis process," I remember being interviewed by one doctor who was particularly "anal." He asked, wondering if he could see a trend in me faking illnesses to get attention, if I had suffered from other diseases. I told him that other than asthma, I never had any previous illnesses.

His reply was monotonic. "That's a good sign. Do you wear glasses?"

I replied that I needed them just for reading.

"Any hearing problems?"

"What?" I replied jokingly.

"Any hear ... Very funny. Okay ... next. How about your bowels – do you move them regularly?"

This gave me great cause for concern. What did he mean by regularly? This, I can assure you, was not a question, or even a thought, that I shared with any of my friends or parents. Therefore, how could I perform a comparison – how could I establish a benchmark to which I could compare and establish what is meant by regularly? I responded with the only reasonable answer. "Yes."

"Are they soft or hard?"

What is he talking about? "What are you talking about?"

He responded with a quizzical look. "Your stool. Are they soft or hard?"

How could I possibly know the answer to this question? It felt like I was taking a biology exam and forgot to study for it. I had no idea it would be this hard ... the questions I mean. "I don't know – is this relevant?"

"Your bowel activity gives us a good insight into your state of overall health. Now, are they soft or hard?"

Intimidated by the question and the process, I succumbed. "I guess they're about average."

"On a scale of 1 to 5?" he persisted.

My god, he's even quantitative about it! He wants me to rate it – assign a number to it, like they do with movies. I was about to object but I quickly realized that he was evaluating not only my answers but also the *way* in which I answered. After all, there are no bounds with middle child syndrome. "I don't know – a three, I guess." Whenever in doubt, always pick the middle.

"Are they light or dark?"

"Dark actually – almost black-like," I said, with astute accuracy.

"Black? Black like the phone?"

"No – but they're shaped like the phone." Now this *is* crazy talk. I never realized one could have a twenty-minute, "educated" conversation about shit. But who am I?

Seeing that I was puzzled and confused, the doctor then turned his questions to other bodily functions. "Please bear with me. How about your bladder? Do you have any problems urinating?"

"No, not at all." That one was easy.

"Do you sleep through the night or do you have to get up to pee?"

"I sleep through the night." I was starting to regain my self-confidence.

"Do you stop after you start or do you have a steady stream?"

It was at that precise moment that I probably confirmed his diagnosis that I was suffering from some sort of *mental problem*. "I don't believe this conversation!" I exploded. "You went to medical school for what must seem like an eternity and all you ask me is if I can go pee-pee or go ca-ca. Doesn't it seem like somewhere down the line you lost sight of your priorities?"

To their credit, my mother, and to some extent, my father, relied on what they knew rather than what they heard from the professionals. They continued to seek help and guidance from their network of friends and contacts. Unfortunately, for two years we sought a proper diagnosis – but to no avail. During the summer of 1971, my health deteriorated to the point that one hot July night I was rushed to emergency (the last recourse when all else fails).

I was operated on the next morning and during the surgery I was diagnosed with Crohn's Disease – an Inflammatory Bowel Disease (IBD). I had over three feet of bowel resected during the surgery and, due to the progressed state of the disease, the recovery process was elongated. In fact, I spent seven full days in the intensive care recovery room before I was stable enough to be transferred to the regular ward.

> *Crohn's Disease is an inflammatory bowel disease (IBD). There is no cure and very little is known today about the main causes or origins. The major symptoms of IBD are chronic pain, cramping, diarrhea, and weight loss. The current treatments involve anti-inflammatory and steroid drug treatment, intravenous feeding and bowel resection surgery. These treatments attempt to lessen the symptoms of these diseases as opposed to treating the cause.*

Approximately six weeks after surgery, while preparing for bed, I noticed that I felt sore in one part of my abdomen and that the incision (or scar) had a very localized redness to it. Unlike my previous hesitancy, I showed my parents immediately. They decided to wait until morning whereupon the redness and soreness were getting worse. My father feared that the surgeons might have left something inside (such as a piece of gauze or other surgical apparatus). I went straight back to emergency (we felt that there was not time to wait for the next follow-up appointment in the surgical clinic). The doctors in the ER called for my surgeon and he rushed in, put me on a gurney and grabbed a scalpel. I was very afraid that he was so intent on getting the gauze (or whatever it was) out that he was going to operate right then and there ... and he did!

There are no nerve endings along scar tissue so as he cut just below the skin to relieve the pressure (and soreness) that was building, I only felt a sense of discomfort. He then routed around in there for a few seconds before pulling out a small piece of black thread! As it turned out, my internal stitches (mending the pieces of intestine) did not dissolve into my system, as they should have over time. The stitches were made out of "cat-gut" and I was apparently allergic to cats – something I would not have known given that cats are not part of my regular food group. Over the next four weeks, as my body released one stitch at a time, the entire incision line, one spot at a time, had opened up and then healed on its own! It was an amazing experience to see the body reject and heal all by itself – I just wish I had been prepared for it!

> *Even in 2004 with the assistance of the global marketplace and international research, there is relatively very little known about it. Further, it is generally accepted that surgery is not a cure – all evidence indicates that the disease will eventually return. In 1971, bowel resection surgery was thought to be the most effective treatment. Now, it's used solely as a treatment of last resort. As we cannot live without a small intestine or bowel, and as the disease will come back and attack a different segment of the bowel, all surgery does is continually reduce the amount of bowel available. The best treatment is to try and reduce the symptoms clinically as much as possible.*

May 22, 1980
Graduation Day, Master of Business Administration

After being diagnosed with Crohn's Disease, my attitude toward everything in life changed. I began to appreciate every moment when I was not sick or in pain. Unfortunately, these were so few that remembering them was not difficult. Whenever I had a choice between doing something now or later, I always picked now because I might not feel as well later. It's a large burden to go through life with, now that I look back; in effect, I was always worried about the next time I'd have to go back into the hospital.

As a result, during my university years, I attempted to take as many courses as possible when I was healthy. I ended up completing my undergraduate courses in two and a half years and did my Masters of Business Administration (MBA) in eleven months and seven days! I completed my last course requirement on December 11, 1979, but did not attend convocation until the following May.

My scheduling tendencies turned out to be very wise in this instance. In early May, I experienced a flare-up of my illness in the form of intestinal bleeding. The bad thing (now that I think about it, there is no good thing) about internal bleeding is that you cannot simply put a band-aid over the cut … you just have to wait for the bleeding to stop. And if it doesn't stop on its own, then surgery is required. After a couple of days of waiting for it to stop at home, I checked into the hospital. Luckily, the bleeding stopped before surgery was required, however, much blood had been lost. I stayed in the hospital for 10 days waiting to regain my strength. During the middle of this stay, I was supposed to graduate. After much pleading, the doctors agreed to provide me with a day pass (almost like a get-out-of-jail card!) so that I could go to convocation and then return. I was so pleased to attend that I didn't notice how weak I'd become – until I tried walking up the stairs of the auditorium!

I completed my convocation duties and returned to the hospital shortly after – happily. No matter what people tell you, the hospital is the best place to be when you're sick! Over my lifetime, I've encountered eight such episodes of internal bleeding – all with no warning. To date, surgery has not been required to stop it.

May 15, 1981 – *Montreal, Quebec*

After my initial surgery in 1971, I began seeing a specialist for the disease – although treatment in the seventies was still more on a reactive rather than a proactive or preventative basis. As a result, very little medical intervention was needed for about ten years other than for the odd bout of bleeding (isn't it funny what we can get used to). Then, again with no warning, I developed a fever with some chronic, low-grade pain in my groin area.

I waited for a couple of days hoping that my condition would automatically get better (don't we all?). With the weekend looming and the fear that no doctor would be found, I contacted my specialist on Friday afternoon (perhaps I *do* have an aversion to the weekend). The news was all bad. I had developed a large abscess in my rectum – an abscess that was about to rupture at any time. Consequently, I needed to be admitted to the hospital to have surgery under general anesthesia that afternoon. I had only one problem – I was to be an usher at a wedding the next afternoon! (One thing that should be clear by now: my timing for the dramatic is impeccable!)

Although my physical well-being was my first concern, the possibility of missing the wedding weighed heavily on my mind. This was a family wedding and I wanted to be part of the ceremony – and part of the photos.

I asked the doctors to postpone the surgery until Sunday or Monday or, at the very least, until after the ceremony on

Saturday. To my surprise, I do believe that the physicians tried very hard to accommodate my desires. They seemed to appreciate the burden of living with Crohn's Disease and wanted to give me a break. Unfortunately, the abscess would not accommodate my wishes and I was forced to have the surgery that day.

With a tremendous amount of guilt, I phoned the groom with the news that I had found something better to do on his wedding day. He was very sympathetic. He was worried when I told him that I had bad news, but was relieved to hear that it had nothing to do with his honeymoon tickets.

Although the doctors could not postpone the surgery, they did their best to do it right away. Unfortunately, a major car accident occurred and I didn't go to the operating room (OR) until 9:30pm that night. After some time in the recovery room, I made it back to my ward shortly after midnight. The doctor advised me that the surgery had gone very well, and, if I had no complications and I felt well enough, I could attend the wedding – but not as an usher. I was advised not to stay on my feet too long.

The morning came fast. Due to my plight, the surgeon ordered less anesthesia than normal and I was able to get over the recuperative process rather quickly. To the amazement of many, myself included, I attended the wedding and performed my usher duties in full (it proved to be too difficult to find someone that could fit into my rented tuxedo). Based on the photos, however, I probably shouldn't have bothered.

March 21, 1983 – *Montreal, Quebec*

After having many things in my life either delayed or cancelled due to illness, I knew that it would take tremendous courage and commitment not let my illness run my life. At this time, I did not truly appreciate how accurate that statement would become.

Similar to the rectal abscess that occurred a couple of years previously, a number of abscesses occurred over a period of the next few years. It became a routine where the abscess would form and I would have to have it drained. These recurrences created lots of scarring and truly made walking almost unbearable, let alone sitting down. I was becoming so much of an expert in this procedure, that even though it required general anesthesia, I handled each of them as an outpatient. One time this occurred during an abnormally busy semester where I was taking doctoral courses and teaching. Because it wasn't an emergency, I was able to schedule the procedure. The best day for me to have the procedure done was on Wednesday – all I had on my calendar was to teach from 8:30am until 11:30am and then from 7pm until 9:30pm. Since I wasn't doing much in the interim, I went to have the procedure done in the afternoon.

The procedure was still considered surgery and as I was under a general anesthesia, I could not have anything to drink after midnight the night before. Therefore, Wednesday morning arrived and I got up showered and went to the University. I taught for 3 hours (with no food or water) and then went to the hospital. I was prepped for the operation and we started the procedure at 1pm. I awoke around 1:45 with a giant pain in the … you get the idea. I then rested and struggled out of the outpatient clinic at 4pm and went to get something to eat – oddly enough, I wasn't that hungry.

I returned to the University that evening and taught my two-and-a-half-hour class before going home and straight to bed. I slept like a baby by the way, waking up every two hours and crying! No one at the University was aware of my predicament – in fact, I was afraid that if anyone had found out, I would get fired for being insane!

August 6, 1987 – *Ottawa, Ontario*

The early eighties were a very difficult time in my life. Crohn's Disease has the tendency to return – even after all the visible signs have been removed from the infected bowel during a resection. This happened a few times and I ended up having two more resection surgeries following the original in 1971 – one in mid-1981 (following the abscess incident) and also in 1985. At this time, the disease had again returned, causing pain, cramping and significant weight loss. As an adult, approximately five feet, ten inches, I weighed only about 115 pounds. Consequently, I was facing my second bowel resection in two years, my third of the decade and fourth overall. As we all have a limited amount of small intestine (about 20 feet), having enough small bowel to absorb sufficient nutrients from food to ensure a healthy life started to become a major concern.

In addition, during the last six years or so, I had recurring Crohn's disease in the rectum. Because of many minor surgeries (like the one in March 1983), the rectum had become ineffective due to the disease and scar tissue. As a result, I had a second consideration – do I have colostomy surgery?

As someone who suffers from IBD, one of the major considerations when leaving the home is – do I know where the nearest washroom is? Bowel urgency is a common occurrence and one that can dominate the thinking to the point of debilitation. Over the years, this consideration became bigger and bigger as my bowel became shorter and the sphincter muscles became increasingly impaired due to conditions described above. In fact, everywhere I went, my first concern was the length of time I could go before needing a washroom; my life choices were being dictated by toilet availability. For the first time in my life, my disease began to take full control of my life – now ordering me in terms of what I could and could not do.

I talked to a surgeon in Montreal who truly believed that I should continue as I had been – performing as little surgery as possible and hoping the disease would "burn itself out" or calm down. Around this time, I agreed to take a job in Ottawa and this afforded me the opportunity to contact another surgeon for a second opinion. The Ottawa doctor was of a completely different mindset. He believed and recommended that I have a colostomy and this would, after recovery and acceptance, give me the confidence to do all of the things I wanted to. Further, he recommended another bowel resection and aggressive medical treatment to try and quiet the disease.

I was now in a very difficult position – two opinions with two completely opposite recommendations. What do I do now? Get a third opinion and let majority rule? It seems like a rather childish way to solve a major problem.

It should be noted that if my new job had not taken me out of town, I might never have received the opinion of a second physician. As patients, we place so much faith in our healthcare system that we can become intimidated by the process and then don't feel comfortable enough to exercise our options. This is the same process that I described in the hockey story, where I respected the coaching fraternity too much and did not forcefully pursue their training and the complete use of the new technology.

I decided to contact a number of friends and they put me in touch with people who had made similar choices in the past. Somehow over time I seemed to know that the most difficult decision was probably the best one (when isn't it?) and decided to go along with the physician in Ottawa – much to the chagrin of my long-time surgeon in Montreal. It has been a decision that I have never regretted.

I found it very frustrating that a framework for support and decision-making was not made available from the hospital or other healthcare providers. As with other health-related decisions, my family and I were really left to ourselves to arrive at a conclusion. It was entirely possible that I could not find people with similar health conditions through my network of contacts. Then what would I have done? What do others do who are less fortunate or less well connected? Where can we turn to get information from a patient's perspective? Where can we go to get information on performance of doctors and hospitals? It could be that the doctor in Ottawa was correct in his recommendation but that another physician was better skilled at doing the actual surgery. How does one – any one – get information of this type? Isn't this something that should be weighed before a final decision is rendered? In other words, we should be able to decide whether or not we will do the procedure as well as have an option of who will perform the procedure.

April 1, 1990 – *Marin County, California*

In late 1988, I moved to the United States for a new job assignment. Unfortunately, my Crohn's Disease came with me and I had a flare-up in the spring of 1990. Being employed, I was automatically enrolled into a Health Maintenance Organization (HMO) associated with my employer – giving me access to a roster of physicians and hospitals. In other words, my healthcare costs would be covered by group insurance – a fact that should not be taken lightly. (*In 2002, over 45 million Americans are not covered by any form of health insurance and a further 55 million are under-insured.*)

After going through the roster of HMO physicians, I found a gastroenterologist that was near my place of work. After the initial medical history update, he provided me with a number of options as to course of treatment and asked me which one *I thought* would be best. My only reaction was: "Excuse me?"

He was somewhat shocked by my response. He stated that it was, after all, my healthcare and I should be active in the decision-making. Since I did not appear to be mentally incapacitated (I must have been having a good day), then I should be active in my healthcare decisions. I readily agreed and then explained to him how all the decisions had been made for me regarding my healthcare in Canada. For example, I was often told what drug to take, when I would have to have surgery and when I could leave the hospital. Now, he was asking me to make the decisions and I was not sure that I was prepared to do it alone. *He assured me that I was not alone.*

Together we decided to start with a course of a new drug that I had not taken before. This seemed to work for a while but conditions got progressively worse after a couple of months. We then agreed that I should enter the hospital for some intravenous feeding. With the weight loss and lack of appetite, my overall health and chemical profile were declining.

In a US hospital, every thing is recorded – and I mean everything! Every time a syringe, IV or band-aid is used, the bar code is taken off the product and put on your chart. At the end of the day, all the bar codes are swiped and a computer printout can then be produced that will illustrate, item by item, a full detailed listing of all the costs that were incurred.

A week after I entered the hospital, my condition had not improved. It appeared that I would be forced to stay in a few more weeks. That would allow for continued intravenous (IV) feeding while I was resting my gut. (This involves the intake of fluids by IV with no food or drink by mouth. The objective is to let the bowel rest and heal itself from the disease – to the point where the patient can start eating again.)

I hate hospitals – in many ways they remind me of prison. You can watch TV but there's no way of getting out – unless it's in the US! I spoke to my doctor and he advised me that I could go home if I wanted. Again, I said, "Excuse me?" – after all this was 1990! He would arrange it with Home Care and I could be set up to do the IV feeding at home. I thought this would be too costly, however, the doctor advised that the $400 a day for Home Care and the medication seem favourable to the insurance companies who would otherwise pay about $2000 a day just for the bed in the hospital. Isn't economics wonderful? I went home the next day.

I stayed on the IV feeding for another three weeks and then managed to successfully return to food. I believe the recuperation period was shorter and more effective because I was at home and was able to relax and recover in familiar surroundings. About a month after discharge, I received a copy of the bill that was sent to my insurance company. It was for seven hospital days, it was forty-two pages in length and it amounted to $27,000 (US, of course).

> *The most important transition in my life occurred during the time that I spent living in the United States, and for this I will be always grateful: I moved from being a patient (or in some ways, a victim) to one of becoming a partner in managing my care (again, in some ways, a survivor). This may not sound like a large transition or distinction, however, just talk to anyone who has a chronic condition and they will tell you the growth is huge. Although I was a very experienced user of the Canadian healthcare system and had sought different opinions and helped make decisions (for example, about whether to have colostomy surgery or not), I had never considered myself to be the person with the final say – i.e., the decision maker – until my time in the States. I guess, before this, I considered my input to be more of a consultant receiving facts on an FYI (for your information) basis – interesting, but you cannot do anything about it. Now, my role was, for the first time, up to me to define.*

At this time, my job saw me returning to Canada for an academic position in Waterloo, Ontario, and I was very interested to see if I could exercise this newfound freedom in the Canadian healthcare system.

December 16, 1991 – *Toronto, Ontario*

The day began like most days in December. Thoughts of the weather, weather-related traffic and long-overdue Christmas shopping pre-occupied my mind. Like most consumers, I feel that the best part of Christmas shopping is when it's all wrapped up, so to speak.

Late this December afternoon, I received a call from my mother. Unlike other calls, she didn't care to talk about the weather or my tardiness regarding shopping for her present. She was all business. She had just visited her doctor – I'm still not sure if it was her GP or a specialist. In any event, she told me that she had just been diagnosed with breast cancer. Her voice sounded distant and detached. It seemed like the longest time before I uttered anything.

Cancer – *cancer* – the big C. We had no family history of cancer. Why would this hit our family now and in this way? Of course, it was not until much later that I realized that every family has no family history of cancer before cancer strikes for the first time.

Once I was able to swallow the large knot in my throat, I began to ask all of the predictable questions. Are they sure? What tests did they do (as if I could make an educated comment on that topic)? Are you going to get another opinion? What are the next steps? Are you going to have surgery? Do you need chemotherapy? How long have you had it – (or the sister question) – can they tell how long you've had it? What are you going to do next?

All the while avoiding the questions that were on both of our minds. Is this life threatening (an answer we all are aware of)? What are your chances of overcoming this? How long do you have?

Once the shock was over and the family had its chance for questions and some answers, you become blatantly aware that you're alone. Yes, there are doctors and support groups but they are not the same as family that will be going through the next steps together. And then the next question becomes very obvious – what are the next steps?

What are the options? Who are the best doctors at treating this type of cancer? Where are these doctors? Who are the best in my province or city? Who are the best in Canada? Who are the best in the world? After all, when your life is on the line, why limit your geography?

Where does one go for this type of information? When something as serious as cancer is diagnosed it's difficult to accept the recommendation of your own doctor without questioning the veracity of his/her conclusion. It's even more difficult to ask your physician for the name of a doctor for a second opinion. We're brought up respecting the medical profession and our doctors in particular. Many of us feel awkward about asking our doctor for the name of a fellow physician for the purpose of checking up on the doctor. Therefore as good Canadians, wanting to avoid confrontation at all cost, we just do not ask.

Even if we do ask for a second opinion or, perhaps, a third, what do we do when the diagnosis differs? When the diagnoses are all the same, the question of treatment and alternatives still must be decided on. It's my belief that a patient support information network must be developed. As patients we have the right to know which doctors or hospitals are the best (and by which measure), what the newest drug research is all about and where we go for research and outcomes information on clinical trials. It's true that there are medical journals that offer information in medical terms, but there is precious little directed at the patient or patient groups.

My mother, with the support of her family, pressured doctors and others to get more information. Eventually she was entered into a research group doing clinical trials and she was part of an experimental group using combined treatment methods. In addition, she had surgery to remove the lump only. It has been over ten years since the diagnosis and selected treatment, and she continues to be cancer-free.

March 4, 1994 – *Montreal, Quebec and Vancouver, BC*

While travelling with the Vancouver Canucks hockey team, I phoned home and learned that my father had passed away suddenly after suffering two heart attacks. My mother had been out all afternoon, and when she returned she called an ambulance to take him to the hospital because he wasn't feeling well and she thought he didn't look well. She followed about a half-hour behind the ambulance (after getting his toiletries and pajamas organized for his expected hospital stay). Unfortunately, she never spoke to him again. I guess sometimes there is nothing even our medical system can do. My mother regrets not getting to say certain things to my father before he died – perhaps it's best to live each moment as if it were our last, after all.

April 1, 1996 – *Toronto, Ontario*

Through the early nineties my Crohn's Disease was fairly quiescent. My weight remained stable and my career became very productive with little interruption due to illness. Before long, however, some of the old symptoms returned.

Once again, I contacted a specialist. Being one of the more difficult cases of IBD, it's not uncommon for my specialists to contact others for consultation. Whereas previously I was told what course of action was next, I have become a very active participant in the decision-making regarding my own health and healthcare.

> *I am not entirely sure what this is due to. It could be the fact that I have had the disease such a long time and no longer want to tolerate being discussed in the third person, or whether my time in the US educated me about the options regarding my participation in my healthcare. In any event, I now have much more control over my treatment.*

The options I face today are the usual ones. First of all, I could have more surgery. This to me, due to short bowel syndrome (a condition that forces long-term intravenous feeding because there is not enough small bowel to absorb enough nutrients to support life), is not a viable option. A second option is to enter the hospital and go on a long-term stretch of IV feeding to rest the gut. (Each time one goes on IV feeding, the recuperation period gets longer.) Unfortunately, IV feeding at home is not as common in Canada as it is in the States. Health insurance companies do not play the same roles across the border, and with government supported healthcare, it becomes a much more difficult exercise in macroeconomics to show the cost benefits of being a patient at home. (Hopefully, with improved information systems in the future, the data can be made available to illustrate the overall benefits of alternative forms of care to the healthcare industry. Otherwise, long overdue change will never take place.)

In the end I decided on a third option, which was to try some new experimental medication. Whereas in the past doctors may have dismissed my willingness to follow non-traditional methods, today they seem willing (at least after much insistence) to try new alternatives. With this medication, due to many potential side effects, I must get a blood test every week to measure liver function. I have accepted this condition and have taken the responsibility for the blood tests and the charting. Every week, I pick up a copy of my blood results and add that to my medical file. I have created an Excel spreadsheet and I graph the results.

Although I'm not sure what all the function results mean, the lab results are very user-friendly. They come with quantitative results and with upper and lower bounds indicating normal levels. I meet with my physician regularly and he monitors the activity. Even though I am not providing any of the medical expertise, I am supplying a visual display of information that assists my doctor's evaluation procedure. In this way, I'm providing value by speeding up the data processing and ensuring data accuracy. This is very similar to the hockey example where the IS allowed the coaches to spend more of their valuable time coaching.

November 22, 1996 – *Kiev, Ukraine*

Shortly after joining the University of Toronto's Faculty of Medicine (in July 1996), I had the opportunity to visit Kiev in Ukraine for a week. The University of Toronto is a member of the Canadian Partners in Health Program for Ukraine. The trip was sponsored by the Canadian Government through the Canadian Society for International Health and funded by the Canadian International Development Agency. As part of the program, faculty members in the Faculty of Medicine (and specifically, the then Department of Health Administration) were going over to Kiev to work with the university in Ukraine, which is beginning to set up a similar program in health administration – and wants to begin the large task of healthcare reform that is long overdue.

I'm not sure whether it was any one thing I saw or sensed or a combination of many things that translated repeatedly into the same word: poor. Without communicating a word, I knew that I had never seen a country, city or neighbourhood in such need of assistance. The problem was, of course, where and how to get started? Education is usually the best place and that's where we began to focus our efforts.

Overall, I was suffering culture shock – perhaps in the truest sense of the term. I had just travelled one third of the way around the world ... and perhaps back in time four decades. I think the most appalling thing about all of this was the lack of hygiene. If we believe that good health and hygiene are related (which I do), then my task of teaching them about health administration was daunting, to say the least.

The first class began ominously. The material that I had sent ahead about three weeks previously had arrived, however, no one had thought to translate it. Obviously, something got lost in the … never mind, you understand. As a result, the lecture that I had prepared based on the preliminary material had to be put aside for another day. As my field of expertise is applied statistics and information systems, I then did an overall introduction into information systems (IS) and then IS in healthcare. With the aid of an interpreter, the class progressed rather well. The students were fabulous and were very interested in learning. The only problems occurred when I told a joke because, after the translation, no one laughed. Then again, maybe that had nothing to do with the translation.

I quickly found out that the material I had sent ahead was probably too advanced and therefore not appropriate for the first set of lectures that the students were to receive in IS. I spent some of the first lecture discussing new hardware and software technologies, but the students had very little exposure to the previous technology, thereby making it extremely difficult for them to appreciate the advancement. To understand and appreciate where one has progressed, there needs to be an understanding of where one has been. I got the feeling early on that my discussions on the state of the art were very similar to describing science fiction. After a while, I became less skeptical and more accepting. The appropriate sense of appreciation could simply not be manufactured.

From the perspective of a university professor in the field of computers and information systems, the week of lectures was a failure. In terms of accomplishing the curriculum, we never even got close. In retrospect, one could probably have anticipated that teaching about new technology would be a waste of time if the audience was not familiar with the old technology. There are very few computers available for them to get the exposure and those that do exist utilize technologies that, in some cases, are up to twenty years old ... or more!

> *The Ukraine students were used to only one style of teaching – the didactic method where the professor professes and the students listen, absorb and regurgitate. It may come as a surprise to many, but the professor does not know everything. There is not just one way to view things. There is not just one way to change things. By introducing the case method (or storytelling), the students, some for the first time, found that their opinions matter, that people were willing to listen to their views. We all have a voice – what good is it if we don't use it? Learning the latest in information systems theory or even learning the case method is not nearly as important as realizing that we all must contribute for the group to succeed. I believe this is important for patients to learn as well.*

As part of my trip, and to assist me in delivering the appropriate focus on new information technology, I had requested a visit to a local hospital or health service centre. On the Thursday morning, I visited a Ministry office building that also housed some pediatric health and social services. Even though my objectives had changed after the beginning of my lectures, I still wanted an appreciation of the role of the government in the Ukrainian healthcare industry.

The official that we met seemed genuinely interested in meeting with me although he appeared to be very defensive at first. When it was communicated (once again, through an interpreter) that I was not here to evaluate or compare, but rather to learn, the mood lightened up. He then served some sparkling wine bottled in Ukraine and began to describe the collection of raw data and statistics completed by his office. As an example of their record keeping ability, he showed me a report that was over 400 pages of *hand-written notes* relating to illnesses stemming from the Chernobyl disaster.

One of his closing comments was that he wanted to emphasize that the government is not only pro-change but is the driving force supporting Healthcare Reform in Ukraine. He was very appreciative of the time I was spending assisting them in developing the curriculum that could be used for their new Master's degree program.

My driver collected me from the hotel on Saturday morning and brought me back to the airport. During this time, I was feeling very run down. I had lost over ten pounds and was still suffering from the after-effects of all of the poor food and eating conditions, the travel and jet lag. Arriving at the departure terminal I had mixed emotions. Firstly, I was very happy to leave. On the other hand, I felt that I had hardly made a dent in the infrastructure; that perhaps my trip had not made a difference. My driver escorted me all the way through the customs process this time. Although I was near complete exhaustion, I was still able to find the duty-free alcohol!

Why have I spent this time discussing my trip to another world? I'm not comparing the North American healthcare system to theirs nor am I threatening that this will happen to all of us if we do not stop our healthcare cuts. Rather, I'm trying to illustrate that we need, as a whole, to get involved with our changes in healthcare. We have a voice, but it's useless if we don't use it. In Ukraine, they do not have our luxuries and they have very little control in shaping their *reform in healthcare. Unlike them, we have a tremendous opportunity – yet we don't seem to want to use it. What we have to do now is to instill some of this urgency into our consciousness **before** our options become too limited.*

October 22, 1999 – *Toronto, Ontario*

Although I've never had any children, I have learned about being a parent and taking responsibility for another person's healthcare through, oddly enough, my dog. Noel was a Yorkshire terrier and died on this day; he was 15 years old plus one day – see, I do have a flare for the dramatic. I know what you're saying: "Here he was making perfect sense in this book until this point; he cannot possibly have any credibility now since he's one of those animal fanatics who treat their pets like children." Well, you may be right. However, I'm not debating that issue here, rather I am illustrating a very valuable lesson that people learn in many ways. I just happened to learn it through the love I had, and the care I shared, for my dog.

At about the age of 12, Noel started developing symptoms of an older dog (which he was). He was gaining weight, very lethargic and constantly drinking water. I took him to my (or his, I'm never quite sure about this) veterinarian and he was puzzled by the sudden change in Noel's condition. We did a number of tests and nothing seemed to come up positive other than the onset of old age. However, perhaps from my own experience (or by using my mother as a role model), I kept insisting that there was something wrong and would not be appeased by the simple "old age" diagnosis. To my satisfaction and to his credit, our (that's probably best) vet kept plugging along at my insistence. Over a period of months, we were able to finally diagnose Noel with Cushing's disease. The cause was unknown, but we knew that he was over-producing adrenaline and that it had many side effects. We then went to see a specialist.

For the next three years (and long after even the most optimistic estimate had passed), Noel continued to be happy and pain free while on the right medication – which I kept on top of (and changed a few times) over this period. You may suggest that I was keeping him alive for my benefit and not his, but once again that's not the topic of debate. The point of this segment is not whether I found some new drug – but rather what I found within me.

As I began lobbying for a better diagnosis and better treatment (in effect, better overall care) for my dog, I found that I was less tentative, more adamant and fully articulate about what I would and would not accept. I was not looking for a miracle or something unreasonable, just the best care. At times, when managing my own care, I would settle or put off an argument for a later time (or maybe to a time when I was feeling better). However, for Noel, there were no trade-offs, no "struggle that was too hard," no "I'll raise that point later." In the end, I was a partner in the decision making with our vet and I truly believe that Noel received the best possible care. When the time came (which it always does, eventually), and there is nothing more you can do, then you must accept that. However, it's quite satisfying in a way to know that there are no doubts, no "what ifs," no "maybe I didn't try hard enough's." And this is all we can ask – to do the best we can do for our loved ones, no matter who they are.

In my research around patient advocacy and the electronic patient record, I discovered that the issues of confidentiality and privacy are two of the major stumbling blocks in moving ahead in a wired world. People are concerned about the breach in security or the wrong group getting access to the record. This information could then be used against them to stop them from getting a job, to take away a driver's license or even to hurt them in a personal relationship. (This is a major issue and must be resolved, as I've stated, through a public debate.) However, one interesting observation is around our children. It seems that as a community, we are more willing to trade off confidentiality against quality of care for our children (and, perhaps, other loved ones although the research is not conclusive in that area). When parents have been asked about entering their children's name in databases or sending electronic files for consultation, there has been very little resistance to change or worry about a breach in security. Unlike, our concern for our own care (and someone finding out about, say, a prescription for a certain medication), as parents, we simply will not risk the best quality of care possible for our child.

Clearly, the perception of technology is the same so therefore there should be resistance – however, there is not. The concern for privacy and security are simply no match compared to the desire to see our child healthy. Parents will do whatever it takes, including the adoption of new technology. As a non-parent, it's hard to understand, or even to hypothesize and then develop the right question to begin the research. Having experienced something similar though, I not only witnessed it but found myself expecting it ... that's what I learned about being a parent from Noel.

The final step is to get people to see their own personal healthcare needs with the same kind of trade-off priorities and to make the same choices for themselves.

December 11, 1999 – *Toronto, Ontario*

This was perhaps the toughest day of my life because of the decisions I had to make regarding my healthcare. Over the last years from 1996 through the end of 1999, my Crohn's Disease was increasing in severity. I have had so many surgeries (some major and some minor) that I lost count after 15 or so (my best guess is more than 20). Therefore, the first option during a flare-up is to try to treat it medically if at all possible. In the fall of 1999, I began developing abdominal abscesses – three of which had to be drained using "interventional radiology."

For the uninitiated, this is simply not fun. I will provide only the highlights. An abscess has formed in the abdomen and the infection must be drained. A major operation could take place. (Unless there is no option, surgery simply cannot be a practical consideration for me. Given the nature of my abdomen and all of the scar tissue, my next major resection will be my last – sentencing me to a life of intravenous feeding.) In order to avoid major surgery then, the first step is to have an ultrasound done on the abdomen to identify (with some precision) the location of the abscess cavity. At that point, a needle is inserted to freeze the area. It should be noted that the area is inflamed (due to the abscess), so to me, it makes very little sense to insert a needle to freeze the area when the area cannot be frozen and the needle causes additional unnecessary pain. After this waste of time, another larger needle is inserted and guided by the ultrasound. If there is any God whatsoever, the needle eventually finds the abscess and the majority of the infection is then drained from the patient. You must use your imagination to understand just how bad the major surgery option must be in order for this hell of a procedure to be considered the "better solution." Basically there is no way to reduce the pain and really no way to send someone else in your place (unfortunately! … and trust me, I did ask if I had to be there).

Just to recap, I had this procedure three times within a couple of months. The question soon became clear: Why was I continuing to develop these abscesses? Further diagnostic imaging revealed a patient (still me) with extremely short small bowel with multiple fistulae (which are tiny holes in the lining of the bowel) that cause many an infection, among other very unpleasant outcomes. Clearly, we needed a solution or I would be having these abscesses drained on a constant basis – and there was no way to guess how many more I could realistically withstand.

A lot of the brainpower at the hospital was called in to consult. Given my own personal health objectives to find the solution that allowed for the best quality of life, we decided to pursue a brand new drug (Remicade, which had not been approved in Canada at that point). This drug has significant potential side effects … and these are the ones we know about. Since it has been around only a short period of time, there is no way of knowing what the long-term effects are or could be.

This was now my major dilemma. Did I stick with more traditional drug therapy which was no longer working, try intravenous feeding for a period of time to see if the abscesses stopped recurring, attempt conservative surgery (which may not end up being conservative at all) or try something so new that no one could truly define all of the possible outcomes? I felt like Captain Kirk being exposed to an exotic strain of virus from a new planet, and "Bones" had an antidote but it had not yet been tested! This was a very difficult decision in my life and, to their credit, my team of doctors let me make the decision alone and said they would whole-heartedly support whatever option I selected. Regardless of the outcome, I respect these physicians more than they will ever know. I decided to follow Captain Kirk; after all, he seemed to live through to the end of each episode.

Although, the doctors were hesitant to "dive into the deep end" with this drug, my severe condition plus my enthusiasm (and one might say insistence) for this option, was critical in facilitating the process of being one of the first in Canada to use this new drug for Crohn's Disease (it has since been approved in Canada for both Crohn's Disease and in the treatment of rheumatoid arthritis).

Since that time, my overall health has showed remarkable improvement. My abscesses have stopped recurring (which means I no longer have a monthly appointment with the "needle from hell") and my bowel absorption has increased. To put it simply, I am now experiencing my best overall health in the last 35 years. Quite remarkable indeed! I know I would not be at this point without this new drug. And I know I would not be on this drug if I had not managed my own healthcare as aggressively as I have learned that I must over the last decade. I am also surrounded by a team of doctors who created a safe environment for me to make these decisions comfortably. I have learned to be my best advocate…and I first experienced this role effectively while managing the care for my dog. He was indeed man's best friend!

February 18, 2004 – *Toronto, Ontario*

When I was first put on the Remicade drug, there was very little knowledge of potential side effects. Now, some five years later, I have more data – and more side effects! Although, it's still too early for completed clinical trials, it appears that the drug either promotes or supports heart disease.

Historically, my heart has been very strong. In fact, I know that I have been able to recover from surgery in short periods of time in part due to a strong heart. This is no longer the case. I was diagnosed with heart disease today.

Heart disease can be very similar to Crohn's disease. Both are chronic and require long term monitoring and management with drugs and with information. In addition, the two are very dissimilar. With Crohn's, patients become aware of the illness and when it will strike. After the onset, managing the disease becomes a matter of work and commitment. With heart disease, however, there usually is no warning and when it strikes it can be fatal. … so if one waits for the next onset, there may be no time to "manage" the illness. Consequently, the patient sits around waiting for the next symptom, which leads to anxiety and a reduction in the body's ability to fight further illness.

In addition to these new concerns, I have also been introduced to a whole new specialty of doctors – the cardiologist. Unfortunately, cardiologists are very "old school" in the sense that they prescribe very specific medication and physical fitness programs. There is usually very little discussion between doctors and patients because they believe that *the* solution is straightforward. It appears to me that cardiologists are very much like surgeons who know what procedure *they want* to have performed. Even though these doctors are usually correct, it would not be a terrible tragedy if they were to spend some *quality time* with the patient in order to find out what they are feeling (emotionally) and whether or not they comprehend the significance of their predicament. This is critical for both the patients *and* the physicians. Cardiologists, surgeons and others may know what is best, but that is not enough because if the patient does not adhere to treatment plans, then the best doctors and drugs cannot help them. It is extremely surprising to me that very few doctors appreciate this fact.

Takeaways from the story

- Ten years ago I would never have been able to write this chapter on my healthcare. Today I can for many reasons: maturity, time needed to reflect and to write, and finding a rationale for sharing it in the first place. The primary constraint to sharing, however, was that I have tried for so long to *avoid* being seen as someone who is sick; after reading my medical history people would most certainly feel sorry for me and that is something that I have tried to escape. If that is the case, then why did I write this book that would make public all my illnesses?

In our society, we have a way of categorizing people so that we can deal with them (and their success), define them, ignore them or evaluate them. I'm not sure why we do this other than to see how we measure up against others. It starts in elementary school (or even before) and it continues throughout life. If someone has achieved more, then we have to find a reason – they were born to a rich family, got very lucky with the stock market and so on. We all seem to do it to some extent. Maybe we do it because we don't want to look deep within ourselves and see that we've let opportunities slip by because we were afraid to try, because we were not paying attention or prepared. Maybe we need to rationalize why other people seem to be happier than we are. However, the simple answer (and I always believe the simple answer) is that we just did not do the best we could have … and that is something that's hard to live with. It's similar to the phenomenon of resistance to change.

We also tend to do this evaluation of people when they are not successful. We see someone who is in a wheelchair, for example, and we feel sorry for them (maybe it's guilt that we're not in the chair) and the situation they're in. We feel pity. This pity, however, does not make that person in the wheelchair (or the person with Crohn's Disease) feel any better, and in some ways, it does just the opposite. They don't want pity because they believe they have not accomplished less or done something wrong. They have faced challenges in their lives, as we all have, and they continue to fight. There is no need for sympathy; there is no need for evaluation or judgment.

We don't need to see how we measure up – we must just be. Unless we all live the exact same life from beginning through every second until the end, how can someone say they did better (or worse) than anyone else (in the ultimate clinical trial, if you will)? This is what I have learned from my illness – that there is no need to evaluate people ... and hence no way for anyone to come up short or feel that they contributed less.

In a lot of ways, I have not discussed my illness in depth to date because I thought it made me look weak or like I did something wrong that caused me to have the illness. Only through meeting a lot of good people and having them share their thoughts and experiences with me have I learned that my illness is not a sign of weakness but rather one of strength. The fact that I have had to overcome a lot of these things and still accomplished everything that I have is a sure testament to that strength, commitment and determination. I am very proud of this fact – and I am proud to write this book on behalf of all patients who have fought through illnesses (some visible and some not) to get to where they are today. In fact, one goal of this book is to make this fight just a little easier, by all of us working together to allow patients to navigate through the health system successfully.

To close this chapter, I want to present the six critical success factors of moving through the technology adoption curve. Here, we present the first three from the perspective of the physician stakeholder group.

1. Amount of resistance to change (i.e., presence of industry experience using the technology)

In the healthcare industry, the main premise of improved information systems is that it will help to increase productivity and improve effectiveness and efficiency. As can be seen from my own healthcare story, physicians have resisted change. Time and again, my healthcare treatment was less than optimal due to poor information systems either on behalf of the clinicians or the hospital staff. This has resulted in delayed recovery and longer than necessary stays in hospital. The rationale is very similar to the primary objection from the credit and loan officers in the banking story: How can technology replace all of my experience and expertise? This is a very difficult argument to oppose and it can only be ultimately defeated through ongoing IT development and deployment success.

2. Amount of training both before and during the transition (or implementation)

While technology consultants are fluent in technology trends, they are not aware of the types of information that healthcare managers would like to have to support, or sometimes to even drive, their decision making. In addition, managers – clinicians, administrators, executives and directors – are not aware of all of the possibilities that technology can offer, either historically or in the immediate and/or near future. The reason for this, of course, is that there has not been a lot of historical success on building information systems in healthcare. Hence, the dialogue between the two parties is often strained. Neither side, normally, is aware of the specific constraints and opportunities that exist on the other side. This communication gap (or void) must be bridged. The only way to do that is to start working together.

Unfortunately, physicians are often over-worked and have no chance to step back and begin working smarter instead of working harder. We must provide support to encourage this work or else it will be very difficult to proceed with further innovation. In my own healthcare management, I relieve some of the burden from my physicians by accessing my own data and charting my progress (hopefully) over time. This allows for a much more thorough interaction when I visit my doctors because they spend more time analyzing the data and results with me rather than trying to accumulate the data and explain it to me. This is very similar to my experience with the NHL coaches: My system allowed them more time to coach and less of a need to be a paper-jockey hustling around looking for files.

3. Amount of buy-in (or contribution during design) from the different stakeholder groups

The initial step in developing any type of computer software or information system should be a complete and accurate determination of user needs and requirements. However, a direct approach seldom produces a response that is complete and useful. "What kind of information would you like?" is rarely a good interview tactic. Managers often do not know what information would be useful or the best way to access or present it. If they did, they would have generated useful information within effective IS long ago. Thus, an indirect approach is often needed in order to be successful.

In management theory, much as been written about the inability of managers to identify their information needs. This is especially true in healthcare where technology can be very intimidating to physicians and staff. Ask any manager what information they would like to have (that they do not have already) – and most are very clear that there are shortcomings to the information they get today – and they would be hard pressed to give you specifics. Most people can tell you what they need once they see it (i.e., with a prototype), but most users have not gone far enough along the development process to think about specific design issues. On the other hand, the IS people are usually very good at developing prototypes, however they need guidance and detailed industry-specific direction. This has been a major stumbling block. Physicians *must* be engaged in the design process in order to ensure that their input is received and their full buy-in is obtained.

The role of the consumer

Over the last decade, consumers, as well as the public in general, have developed an increased demand for better information and better service. This information must be accessible, accurate and easily understood; and if consumers do not get it directly from the source, they will find other ways to obtain what they need to know. Moreover, changing technology has had a tremendous impact in all areas of society. In health, the growth in computer functionality and bandwidth has already begun to have a dramatic effect.

In the near future, information on best practices will be readily available to physicians through digital libraries. Patients will be able to schedule their own appointments and organize all of their procedures to fit their busy lives. Information technology will be able to reach patients in remote areas that previously could not be treated very efficiently or effectively. Ultimately, technology will provide a methodology to overcome access and utilization discrepancies throughout our society. Consumers, regardless of social class and income, will be able to learn more about illness and health promotion – resulting in access to information becoming a significant determinant of health.

One necessary condition for this consumer and technological maturity is a well-versed and accepted strategic direction for healthcare. Investment in technology cannot take place without first understanding the health delivery system and the information requirements for the future.

It's difficult to conceive of all of the benefits that information technology will provide, as the change throughout healthcare will be staggering. It is anticipated that information technology, when implemented in an integrated and effective manner, will even change the nature of medical care itself. For example, the patient armed with health, medical and system information, will indeed become a more active decision maker. The obstacle impeding this revolution to date (a revolution that began long ago in other industries) is the lack of accessible information made easily available to patients. However, once this becomes more of a reality, the revolution will occur throughout health ... and the consumer will demand it.

4. Level of consumer (or end-user) influence during early stages of adoption

The only area where patients seem to be voicing themselves is on the Internet with patient support groups and message boards. Health Web sites are some of the most popular sites all around the world. Patients are finding a way to get to information. However, this has *not*, at least to date, been facilitated by the healthcare field – we have had to do it by going around the system or the industry.

As patients become more active participants in the decision-making process, there must be an increased demand for access to their own personal health information. Studies have found that patients are willing to use electronic media for education, assistance in decision-making and as a source of personal health information.

I have shown how I have found ways to get access to my health information so that I can be an integral part of the decision-making team. It's only at this point that the true effect of the educated patient (i.e., consumer in healthcare) will be realized.

Performance Measurement

As in other industries, health professionals need to be able to measure what resources they are using to provide quality of care, at what cost, and to what end – and the effectiveness of that care. Moreover, there are many different levels of detail required for many different health stakeholders: the kind of information required by a department manager differs considerably from the kind of information required by a Board of Trustees. In addition, the focus of the information could be varied: from a technical point of view when assessing the value of a treatment, to the customer's point of view when assessing the value of that same treatment. As well, the scope of information may range from a department level or functional focus to a community-wide process focus.

A complete and exhaustive listing of the outcomes or benefits is needed to help illustrate the importance of electronic health or patient records and the significance of investment.

Individual Patient Benefits:

1. Patients able to access their own record across providers (thereby eliminating the current lack of an integrated patient record) which can now form majority of the decision support needed to interact more effectively with the health system
2. Patients able to refer to their own family history
3. Physicians able to examine complete, accurate profile of patient due to new consistency in data capture and data files within providers

4. Physicians able to get immediate access to patient history
5. A reduction in the current duplication of tests or treatments
6. A way to examine utilization of system for forecasting
7. Will provide an environment for accountability to the public
8. Will allow for easier management of the system (i.e., fraud, inconsistent patterns)
9. Will result in lower research costs due to easier access to accurate data
10. Will result in more research involving sophisticated data analysis.

Health System Benefits:

1. Patients will be able to review system performance
2. Patients will be able to examine options and select the best provider (e.g., hospital, doctors) for themselves
3. Patients will be able to schedule appointments for multiple procedures to gain efficiencies
4. Patients will have access to better and more relevant information (as opposed to what is currently available on the Web)
5. Physicians will be able track patients to ensure they comply with treatment
6. Physicians will be able to analyze groups of patients for potential illness or reactions
7. With better information and more efficient processes, there will be reduction in overall system

cost, e.g., reduction LOS, lower use of diagnostic imaging and other tests, fewer lab requests, lower home care utilization

8. Improved community care services as information will travel ahead of the patient (instead of either with the patient or not at all)

9. More research in health services will be made easier and less costly, driving up evidence-based decision making

10. Physicians and other providers will be able to provide better care resulting in improved effectiveness – i.e., better health outcomes.

In the end, we must translate these "benefits" into specific metrics so that we can effectively measure the health system's performance and growth over time.

5. Level of the effective reporting on the status of the outcome measures during and post-implementation

Most strategic investment decisions incorporate a business case evaluation (as we illustrated in the banking story) where all of the future benefits are weighed against current and future costs. The objective, of course, is to only invest in initiatives that have more benefits than costs. During the development of these types of business cases, the accurate evaluation of benefits and of costs is of utmost importance. Incorrectly calculating the costs or the timing of the benefits may lead to decisions that differ from optimal. Business cases for initiatives surrounding new technology or new information systems (IS) are no different.

Although cost components of technology are usually straightforward, such as with the hardware, programming and the like, the benefits, on the other hand, are extremely difficult to measure. How do you put a price tag on the ability of someone to do their job better; or how do you calculate people enjoying their jobs more and, consequently, being more effective? What is needed is the ability to create standards of measures of performance such that the resulting benefits of increased efficiency and effectiveness can begin to be evaluated. Many state, in arguments resisting change: "Why do we need change, things are going well?" Of course, my response to that challenge is: "Going well compared to what?" How much better could things be if we adopted new strategies, new designs, new systems? Since we do not have the facts to answer these questions, we must investigate them further. The truth can only be found when we are looking for it and want to see it.

6. Level of effectiveness in dealing with good or bad fortune

As patients move to this more self-reliant role in the management of their health, the requirement of individual health information in electronic format becomes obvious. Otherwise, if we remain in a paper-health-record world, the data will remain inaccessible by patients. At a large academic health science centre in Toronto, a research team was engaged in one of the first patient-centred research efforts of its kind. The project engaged patients as stakeholders by asking them to design, using innovative technology, an effective electronic patient record interface.

The project employs a systematic patient-centered, iterative approach to system design, development and evaluation. The only real hurdle has been that many physicians were skeptical about the value of patients accessing their own records and how the patients would react. The physicians worried about increased workload involved in handling extra questions, and about how patients would react emotionally when they accessed their record. Further, there was serious concern over the integrity and security of the data emanating from the many people with remote access to active health records. In fact, the major obstacle was convincing the doctors that there was a need at all (or even the demand) to access records remotely and, thereby, electronically. This battle was going very slowly.

In early 2003, SARS (Severe Acute Respiratory Syndrome) hit Toronto and had a major impact on the healthcare community. Doctors who entered hospitals to treat patients were exposed to the potential of a forced quarantine, the effects of the virus, or both. Suddenly, doctors and other clinicians saw tremendous benefit to being able to access records and all sorts of patient and health information remotely. The research project continues, with a partnership of both clinicians and patients potentially remotely and electronically accessing patient records.

Clearly, there are events in life that are unpredictable – some which will have a positive effect and some which will have a negative effect. Being able to take advantage of both types of outcomes will increase the likelihood of success for any project. In this story, a number of months of further struggle were eliminated due to the intervention of a "break" – one that had an extremely negative impact on the healthcare service delivery sector, but which created an outcome that may benefit the industry for years down the road.

Finally, as in the other stories, there is a need to make the link between the new technology and the old ways of doing things. In this case, the link was to illustrate to the doctors that the issues relating to patient access to medical records are exactly the same as they are for physician access. The SARS outbreak was a way for many clinicians to witness first-hand the frustration of not being able to access the information needed to accomplish goals.

"Patients must not be afraid of getting to know their health care network and their health care network needs to do more to outreach to them. After all, is it not things we don't know which end up harming us and costing us the most?"

Huguette Agnes Burroughs,
journalist and patient.

"Because the only thing worse than something happening is knowing that it could have been prevented. Speak up if you have questions or concerns and don't be shy about asking your doctor or nurse for more information from reliable sources. Good health professionals value the relationships they have with their patients."

United Health Foundation
(www.unitedhealthfoundation.org)

CHAPTER SEVEN

The need for an
IS vision statement

Healthcare is evolving rapidly in order to deal with both financial realities and ongoing scientific progress. To ensure that this evolution results in a system that provides the highest quality, there is an increasing need to better understand and manage healthcare. In some detail, health professionals, across the continuum of care, need to be able to measure the resources they are using to provide quality of care, at what cost, and to what end – and the effectiveness of that care. Well-developed information systems are crucial to providing timely, accurate and comprehensive information about costs, quality, utilization, workload, outcomes and satisfaction. The need for electronic communication and networking is paramount.

Unfortunately, healthcare providers currently lack effective information systems. In fact, there is very little agreement on what data we have, what information is missing, what information is indeed needed and what system is needed to generate this support. Consequently, recent initiatives to address the IS problem have failed for a number of reasons which are quite complicated and complex.

In order to develop organizational strategy and related objectives, a Healthcare Information Systems Vision Statement (HISVS) is of paramount importance. It is my intent here to propose such a Vision Statement. Like most of these statements, however, many arguments and competing theories can, and most likely will, be suggested and debated. That being said, I do not believe that we can have a constructive discourse on a Vision without first developing a starting point. Therefore, it is with this spirit of discussion and consensus that I propose the following Health Vision Statement. In order to guide us there, I first present a series of premises, many of which should be readily accepted.

Premise One:
Times have changed

This may not appear to be all that insightful, at first glance, but this premise contains very important building blocks for a vision. We are no longer in an era where businesses and governments tell people what to do and when. The rise in consumerism has created the demand from the public for better information and better service. We no longer live in a society where people are satisfied to get their cash in person from only one branch of one bank between the hours of 10 am and 3 pm, Monday through Friday. We live in an "MTV" world where people get bored and flip the channel if they don't see what they like within 15 seconds (and sometimes, even less than that). The public wants information in the way they want it, when they want it; and companies that can deliver it, (whether it's by using the Internet or some other delivery channel), will be successful.

We have rapidly progressed through the Information Age into a "Knowledge Era." Information that is meaningless to consumers has no value. Organizations that can make infor-

mation relevant (i.e., knowledge) are the ones that will experience tremendous growth. The last twenty years has seen
some fantastic growth in technological capabilities and companies that were integral parts of that growth have made
incredible fortunes. In the next twenty years, the industries that
will be successful will be the ones that can take advantage of
that technology and deliver pertinent information, which is
targeted knowledge down to the individual consumer. Up until
today, the focus has been on bandwidth or the size of the
message; the focus of tomorrow will be on the content or the
message itself.

Times have indeed changed!

Premise Two:
Patients are at the centre of healthcare

Again, this may seem trivial. We've seen many Hospital
Mission statements echoing this same message – changing to
a more patient-centred care. However, I do not believe that
this message has been firmly understood or appreciated.
Without the patient, there is no need for healthcare professionals. The patient is the one constant throughout all of the
health delivery system.

When this premise is combined with the first one, it
becomes fairly obvious that the patients, in the near future,
will begin to demand better health information. To emphasize,
I do not believe that the average consumer is concerned with
the specific care they would receive in hospitals today. There
have been many stories written about our system in decay
throughout the media, but it is my belief that the public is not
unhappy about the system. In the Ontario Hospital Association

Report Card (1999), a number of findings substantiate this point. For instance, 76.4% of patients rated their overall quality of care to be excellent (OHA, 1999, p.62). In addition, 53.9% of patients stated their satisfaction level with their hospital outcome was excellen (OHA, 1999, p.66). What patients do want, however, and will demand, is better information about the system, about who performs what services and about how well they do it. Answers to these questions will allow consumers to make informed decisions surrounding services.

Patients, as opposed to consumers, want different information. (I refer to a consumer as someone who uses the health system very infrequently, has no chronic conditions, and hence, has had no or little sporadic interaction with the system; patients, on the other hand, are in much more frequent contact with the system, perhaps have chronic conditions, and often rely on the system to achieve their own lifestyle expectations.) Patients want access to their own patient record, and they want to be able to understand what it is they're reading. In addition, they want to know more about their illness or disease and they want information on treatment options and success rates. Often, they would like to get in touch with other patients to exchange experience and to get advice. After all, it's only when they interact with other patients that they get real information about what they are going, or will go, through.

Premise Three:
Ultimately, patients are the decision makers

When patients are faced with difficult healthcare questions, they seek advice from their doctor(s), other health professionals, and their own personal network. Even though the physician will provide the best medical support, ultimately it is the patient who has to decide whether they want this drug treatment or that surgery. It's understood that not all patients may have the maturity or cognitive ability to comprehend the decisions that they have to make. Many have used this argument to defeat premise 3; but, in actuality, this rebuttal only applies to a small percentage – perhaps, conservatively, twenty percent of our population. The remaining eighty percent have the ability and the right to make their own decisions. What they lack is the medical background needed to facilitate all the information and to process it in order to make an informed choice.

It is my belief that in the healthcare system of the future, we will see physicians and other professionals act as advisors to patients rather than the old model where patients are told what to do (more of a "guide on the side"). Gone will be the day where patients will feel that they are not free to question facts or options.

Premise Four:
Decision makers need information

Once again, this seems rather straightforward. It's well understood in information theory and in the decision analysis literature that decision makers need information to assist in making any decision. If we apply this premise to Premise 3 above, then it becomes clear that we must get the critical information to the patient in order for them to make informed decisions. This means that the focal point of the healthcare system of the future must be around the patient record since that is the only point where all the data resides. In order to move the data and information around efficiently, it's obvious as well that this record will have to be in electronic form – hence the need to develop Electronic Patient (or Health) Records (EPRs or EHRs).

Premise Five:
Our healthcare delivery system is fragmented.

Patients do not receive all of their care and treatment in one location. They receive treatment in doctors' offices, clinics, different hospitals and even in their home. Not only the realities of today but also the delivery design of the future, creating a patient record that contains all relevant health data as described in Premise 4 in one place will not be easy.

The hospital system over the last few years has spent millions of dollars building internal information systems using the latest technologies. Unfortunately, they have not all implemented the same systems. Further, the focus has primarily been on internal connectivity within each hospital, leaving all external networking as a secondary objective due to a lack of understanding of where the system was/is headed (i.e., no vision statement). To paraphrase from Lewis Carroll's *Alice's Adventures in Wonderland*, if you don't know where you are headed, then any road will take you there!

VISION STATEMENT

If the patient is going to be making all of his/her decisions and since the information from data that has to be analyzed is scattered all over the healthcare system, then we must be able to link all of this data together in order to achieve the information support that is needed. This condition must be accepted if we are ever to gain benefit from information technology in healthcare.

It should be emphasized that the key word in the above vision statement is "link." As stated, many health organizations have already spent significant resources in developing their own internal systems. Many have gone through their own growing pains and would resist any suggestion to re-develop and/or re-implement. It is just not feasible (i.e., cost effective) to put all of this to one side and begin anew. In fact, different hospitals testing different software and hardware configurations allow for sound comparison and evaluation, which may lead, hopefully, to improved system designs for second generation IS development.

Therefore, an interface must be developed that would allow systems of many different structures and functionality to operate effectively – independent yet integrated with one another. This type of interface, at least initially, would be read-only in nature. The rationale for this is the many different databases and data capture processes that are in place today in Ontario hospitals. Any project that would have full data integration as a necessary condition for implementation would take years to complete.

If systems do not need to have data integration across all computer systems, then there must be a common data structure that is agreed to, and becomes standardized, when organizations move data around through a secured network. In other words, when computers talk to one another, there *must* be a layout of the data (referred to herein as a Health Data Packet or HDP) that would be used consistently by all providers. The specific content within the HDP should contain identifying data as well and pertinent medical information, presumably at a very high level. (The intent at this phase is not to design the HDP but rather to elaborate on the concept; it is understood that many varied stakeholder representatives would work together to identify the specific data elements within the HDP.)

One possible outcome of the HDP is that all hospitals, and other providers, will be able to link with each other directly in order to gain access to information in much the same way they can today through the Internet to access pages of a read-only nature. This option, however, has limitations. The most significant is that individual hospitals, when dealing with a patient, will only know to go to a second hospital, or to any other provider, to gain read-only access if the patient advises them. In emergency cases, this information may not always be available. Hence, there will be no one single point of access that could ensure that nothing was overlooked. With this structure there still will be no single place where a patient can go to get a comprehensive overview of their medical status.

Consequently, I recommend a separate organizational entity whose full time mandate is to get the HDP from all health providers (presumably online) and then re-organize the data so that there is real-time access to comprehensive individual patient records. This type of structure is currently used in the banking industry for their credit bureau files and has been successfully operational (and extremely profitable) for decades. Credit bureaus have evolved over time and have seen their functionality improve to the point where files are returned in approximately two to three seconds (as we have seen in chapter five in the banking story). The hardest part of maintaining their central linking function is the development of algorithms used to reconfigure data layouts from individual creditors into a layout that matches their database.

In health, this requirement could be eliminated through the creation of the HDP – which means that all data accessed will already be in a common format. It must be emphasized that there will be no centralized database created per se; all of the data will be integrated virtually only when requested. The only data that would be kept in a centralized location is the complete set of links that any one patient has across all health service providers. Otherwise, the data remain in their current location under the individual organization's security surveillance and within operational firewalls.

On a go-forward basis, there are many technology companies that would be extremely interested in developing the technology to manage such a "health bank" or virtual database of linkages. For this to work, however, we must create an organization that would be responsible for the operation of this system and accountable to the people. Whether this should be done on a national level or not is debatable, however for our discussion, I will refer to this simply as the HealthBank (HB). Consequently, when patients interface with the health system, they, or a designated health provider, will presumably contact the HB and access the virtual EPR created from the HDPs from all contributors. It will be the responsibility of the HB to identify the complete list of linkages that any one person has throughout the national health system.

Further, the EPR, in addition to providing demographic and critical health information, will contain pointers to the specific contributing health providers indicating where more detailed data and information can be found if so needed. The hospitals or other providers would then communicate to the inquiring source to determine the best way to transmit this more detailed follow-up information.

This vision of a central link using an index-pointer repository of the type described herein will address the following:

- Lack of an integrated patient record
- Duplication of tests or treatments
- Inconsistent data capture and data files within providers
- Inability to access information in a timely manner
- Costly infrastructure to get all hospitals operating on the same system.

In addition to providing these benefits (see below for a more comprehensive list), research and health system evaluation will be greatly assisted. The HB would provide data for any research relating to utilization, health outcomes or best practices. As well, the ministries of health across the country could use some of the data to monitor utilization, estimate system costs and to examine extraordinary events.

One final comment that should be addressed is the need for a unique patient identifier. There is no way to feasibly create a solution of the type described here without a unique number to match patient information from various databases and ensure 100% accuracy. As with all of the concepts presented here, the details can only be resolved and finalized through public education and debate.

HOW DOES THIS VISION ASSIST
IN PATIENT DECISION-MAKING?

The key outcome of the Vision as presented here is that the patient will be able to access an integrated electronic patient record to assist in the management of their care. Our thesis is that patients, once exposed to the benefits of the EPR will be one of the strongest advocates for change and will work with their health service providers to overcome the drawbacks (e.g., potential security risks) in order to access the benefits. However, patients must develop a comprehensive understanding of all benefits if they are to support the use of an EPR.

As such, concerted efforts should be made to comply with design principles based on human-computer interaction research. Poor design can complicate the navigational process for patients and clinicians, and increase demand on their attention, perception, language, and memory. By acknowledging these constraints, the structural design of the EPR should aim to match existing user workflow, follow established standards, accommodate flexibility, and recognize human limits. Well-designed electronic records should focus the viewer's attention on the data. The information should be presented in an easily navigable structure and comprehensible format.

"One of the most radical steps toward consumer empowerment will involve making the
electronic health records (at least parts of them)
available to consumers on the Internet. Once
this occurs, consumers will be able to do 'on-line
doctoring', just like they do 'on-line banking'
and 'on-line shopping' today.

Dr. Gunther Eysenbach,
Head, Research Unit for Cybermedicine and eHealth,
University of Heidelberg, Germany.

CHAPTER EIGHT

A series of four treatments

In this chapter, I outline four very straightforward objectives or treatments for the healthcare industry that emanate directly from the presentation and arguments made throughout this book. It is my belief that the attainment of these objectives presented as "prescriptions" and the milestones therein (many of which migrate across objectives) will form the backbone of a new, truly patient-centered healthcare system of the future!

THE SYMPTOMS

Perhaps the most frustrating of all experiences patients have with healthcare professionals is the lack of communication and continuity. Consider the case where we see only one physician. We would expect that physician to have access to all of the history that we have had with him or her. Some physicians are able to perform much of this continuity through their own memory – which is very comforting – without even referring to their own notes. In addition, we expect this physician to have access to all of the test results that had been ordered such as blood tests, x-rays and the like. Even if the x-rays were not in the physician's office, we would expect the results to be available in summary form. If we were to go to this doctor's office for a follow-up visit, we would be very disappointed if the physician were unable to access the results or even failed to recall ordering the results. Further, we would be very suspicious of a physician's ability to manage our healthcare if he/she were unable to specifically recall the rationale for the exact prescriptions that we were given during the last appointment visit.

Now consider the case where we see our general practitioner on one visit and then are referred to a specialist who we visit on the second appointment. In this scenario we would expect there to be discontinuity of care. We would expect that the specialist would not know, or be able to even access, our extensive health history and would, in all likelihood, be unaware of what medicines we are on or have been on in the past to treat the current ailment. Moreover, it would be very difficult for the specialist to access results or actual copies of x-rays, ultrasound tests and the like.

The only way for this specialist, in most cases, to have this type of information is if we, the patients, carried our own patient file, record or chart, from the first doctor's office with us until the time when we visit the second doctor. Often, this method of information transportation is not viable. This usually results in longer patient interviews with the specialist, redoing tests, some which can be very uncomfortable, uncertainty in prescription history, and a less than optimal course of treatment due to ineffective and inefficient method of information transfer.

One of the two scenarios described above is a stretching of the truth or an exaggeration of current capabilities; unfortunately, it is the first one. Since most of us are unfamiliar with how information is passed along in the medical profession, we believe that the cases described are fairly reflective of what happens. The fact is that our faith in the system is very much misplaced, even in the case where we see only one physician, even when that physician is our general practitioner and even when this person is the one who has managed our care for a long period of time.

The truth is that, other than keeping paper records in a filing cabinet in his/her office, one doctor is not any more likely to have access to a complete medical record (test work, surgery results, consultation notes from another specialist/ physician) than two or more doctors. The reason is that there is no information transfer system, there are no standards, there is no protocol. There is no single, comprehensive health or patient record.

Had the health field advanced at the same rate as the financial services industry, we would have electronic access to our health record, at any time, at any hospital, at any place. Further, we could access multiple databases, perhaps through computer software, in order to get test results such as blood tests for pregnancy, verify prescription history at the local pharmacy and evaluate performance measures for a number of physicians at a specific hospital that we might be considering for future treatment.

Contents within an EPR
The first stage in the process of creating more effective information systems in healthcare is the design and development of a database of patient care data. Healthcare pertains to providing care to patients and, as such, the database must begin there. After the successful implementation of such a database, efforts can then begin on a more comprehensive

data-set which would include financial, organizational, physician and patient-focused data. If we attempt to develop all aspects of a comprehensive database at once, we risk diffusion of effort and early mistakes which may be impossible to overcome in later stages.

In the end, any doctor, from any location will be able to access your complete and accurate health record. This will enable the practitioner to offer the most effective care. It will not matter if you have never seen the physician before (as in an emergency room visit) or you see the general practitioner that you've been seeing your entire life, the level, accuracy and completeness of the data will be consistent. This will reduce ineffective and inconsistent care, repeated and needless tests, and patient frustration with the overall system.

A final goal is to allow the patient to access his or her own file at least on a read-only basis. This will require controls for accessibility, privacy and confidentiality, all of which are issues that are described later in this book. Access to one's own file can allow for updating incorrect information, verifying prescription usage and assisting with the promotion and implementation of all issues pertaining to a consumer-focused healthcare system where the customers become responsible for managing their own healthcare.

The short-term goals of this book include determining the type and scope of the information that would be useful to healthcare providers and decision makers, as well as the usefulness of making this information accessible to others in the healthcare community and the factors that would inhibit such a process of sharing. Further evolution will necessitate the development of a methodology for establishing a database of health delivery data – including both cost and health performance measures. Hospitals and other healthcare services in local regions could be used to validate the methodology and establish the initial data pool. This validation process should include both the development of measurements and the creation of feasible standards or benchmarks. Once the validation is completed, the database will be expanded through the inclusion of data from other interested hospitals and healthcare delivery centres.

Ultimately, the long-term solution focuses on the development of a framework for an electronic patient health record. By concentrating continuous improvement efforts on database design, a foundation can be properly created to establish long term, overall system performance improvement. As such, researchers have indicated that a continuous, lifetime, personal medical record would allow better assessment of the cost-effectiveness of many preventative, diagnostic, and therapeutic activities. Such a record would also benefit the patient by ensuring consistent, integrated care and ease of transition between healthcare institutions and providers – a need that definitely exists.

If health administrators and care givers (across all providers in a community) knew *which* of their activities were having a positive impact on the quality of their patients' lives, if they knew *how* their activities were impacting that quality and by *how much*, then those administrators and care givers would be able to reallocate current resources to achieve more. Or perhaps they could maintain the current level of service with fewer resources. In addition, incorporating a collaborative attitude toward information management throughout the community could affect increased efficiencies and improve quality of care. Information is the key to saving our healthcare system, more and better information than is currently available.

Systems design

The new world of electronic connectivity in healthcare (eHealth Innovation) will enable long term and other healthcare agencies to re-engineer and create effective service delivery plans. Currently, a client requiring more than one service is repeatedly asked the same questions and each agency does their own assessment and creates duplicate files. The information is not shared and the client experiences first hand the disjointedness of the system. A centralized intake function connected to an effective information system would allow for the reduction in duplicate information, a timely transfer of information between agencies, and a reduction in staff hours required to assess and document much of the same information. Information that is obtained then represents a value-added benefit. Professionals performing specialized assessments are able to focus time on their particular discipline and have the benefit of the previous assessments and data contained in the client's file.

> By eHealth Innovation we mean the conceptualization, design, development, application and evaluation of new ways of using existing or emerging Information and Communication Technologies (ICTs) in the health sector. This concept goes beyond pure technological considerations. eHealth Innovation includes the effects of ICTs on society, the culture of health and health care in general, and in particular its effects on access to health information and services, as well as to the advanced medical technologies themselves. The common foundation for all of these disciplines is Information Management.

The increasing availability of detailed health-related information across the Internet is resulting in an urgent need to study the quality and impact of this information and also to detail the impact that this might have on the physician-patient relationship.

Fragmentation of service

If a doctor's office or a clinic were to send a patient to a large hospital, perhaps in a different town or city, the patient would have to carry his/her records with them. There really is no other option (other than perhaps faxing multiple pages). Networking, through the incorporation of the unique patient identifier, would facilitate this process by allowing for one comprehensive and effective information system to be developed. There would then be standards for both data capture and for data transmission. Consequently, we must address the need for and the implementation of a UPI in this country.

Lack of performance measures

Moreover, there are no standard measures for performance, whether it deals with patient survival for experimental surgery, whether it ranks doctor performance with respect to waiting in his/her office for appointments, or in rating hospital food during inpatient stays. There just are no measures. However, health system reporting must become more effective through better system evaluation.

Centralized health data versus other configurations

Certainly, an effective health information system consisting of health data from many sources must be integrated at some level. Otherwise, the disjointedness, redundancy and fragmentation that exist today would continue except that it would be electronic (and access time to incomplete data would be reduced). However, the only time a complete, efficient database is needed is during a treatment episode or inquiry. At that time, a virtual centralized record can be constructed, almost instantly, with immediate subsequent computerized inquiries to the multiple sites involved. With the appropriate software and algorithms, redundancies can be removed and a comprehensive record provided within seconds.

In short, many different format-types and structures, some of which have been suggested above, can be effective; that there is no one optimal configuration. It should be noted that much of the final selection would rely on the cooperation and the technology available to all of the partners in the systems or network. Agreeing to, and accepting the philosophy of, a comprehensive electronic patient record is much more critical than the actual data location.

All of these areas presented above (and many more) require the involvement from the patient community in order to ensure effective design and development. Patients must be a part of the solution and decision process!

THE DIAGNOSIS

The health industry must be in step with information system, service levels and the customer-centred focus that has been attained in many other industries in this new millennium.

Patient involvement in this process is critical in order to ensure the effective completion of this process. From a patient perspective, some of the direct benefits as we move to a more effective electronic health world will be:

- Availability when live contacts are busy or not available
- Consistency in gathering and dispensing information
- Customized instruction
- Patient privacy protection and avoidance of embarrassment
- Apt use of learning, feedback and reinforcement
- Access performance measures; track improved outcomes.

Unfortunately, the health industry has had a completely different focus from that of other industries. In banking, for example, the customer drives the service, not the bank teller or even the manager. With competition just across the street, whatever the customer wants (within reason), the customer gets. Therefore, whenever innovation or technological advancement, as in the development of information systems, can be used for competitive advantage, the banks (i.e., private industry, are very willing to adopt change to challenge the system and attract the customer.

In healthcare, however, the doctors, to date, drive the industry, not the patients. Therefore, the focus of change has been on technological advancement for diagnostic testing and procedures, such as MRIs (magnetic resonance imaging), ultrasounds and laprascopic surgery, areas that can improve the doctors' delivery of care. In these types of areas, there has been a tremendous technological revolution, sometimes dramatically changing the way we deliver healthcare. This is not to say that the patient has not benefited from this doctor-patient focus. For example, it is now possible to have abdominal surgery, such as gall bladder surgery and removal, and be back to work within 14 days where traditionally patients had in-hospitals stays of 7 to 10 days, depending on complications or post-operative infections, with somewhere from a four to six week recuperation at home.

The focus clearly has been on improving care for patients. The focus, however, has *not* been on improving information or communication *to* the patients. In addition, the concentration of research has been on treating a patient – on an individual basis or individual disease, not on patients as an entity. Therefore, communication within this industry, between doctor and patient, between hospital and doctor, between ministry and doctor, or ministry and hospital has never really been accomplished. As we progress with further belt-tightening cost reductions, these levels of information are critical.

Since there has been very little successful adoption of information technology throughout healthcare, the resistance to change factor has played a huge role for both physicians and patients. This has led to episodic IT adoption with one of the main contributing factors to its poor success rate being a lack of stakeholder involvement. In building information systems, all users have to be involved, or the system gets created ineffectively. If all users do not have input, then there will be some criteria that will not be heard and hence the system that will be developed will not address all of the users' needs. This results in resentment and lack of adoption.

Let me illustrate using the following story.

One day, a very rich and successful businessman approached an architect to design a new home that he wanted to build in the secluded mountains overlooking the great lakes of Minnesota. When the businessman asked about when the architect would consult him on his wants and objectives for the new home, the architect said that he had a better way to design homes – he just observed the customer and improved the design of the present home environment, so to speak. That seemed to satisfy the businessman, as he was very supportive of innovation.

When the house was built, the businessman was very surprised to find that the architect had put the refrigerator in the TV room. When asked, the architect stated, "Every time you were watching TV you went repeatedly to the kitchen to retrieve items from the fridge; in fact, you spend relatively little time in the kitchen at all." It just made sense to me to move the refrigerator into the TV room.

Obviously, only so much can be gleaned through observation alone!

Finally, there has been little, at least until just recently, accomplished in establishing performance metrics to evaluate the healthcare system in general. Therefore, relating an improvement in health outcomes (if there is one) back to IT investment has been extremely difficult. Consequently, and unfortunately, communication on performance metrics during or after the implementation is only a theoretical construct in today's healthcare environment.

THE TREATMENTS

Prescription One
Begin to realize the role that information systems can play

The acceptance of the role of information systems and technology as an integral component of a decentralized model, delivering a seamless continuum of care, must be recognized. Once the hurdle of recognizing the need for information systems has been overcome, the next step is to focus on the form that information must take to be useful. Years of improper system design and long delays resulting in inaccessibility of the information has led to a perception that computerization only accomplishes the further cluttering of desks and offices within organizations.

The theory of Information Systems concentrates on getting the right information at the right time in the right format to the right user. The development of information systems, requires focus on organizational objectives, design and dynamics as much as it requires focus on the procurement of the most appropriate hardware and software. Today, the concentration on issues pertaining to computer-based systems is often incorrectly emphasized. Computers play an integral role in the development and operation of information systems, however, the computer-related functions should primarily be supporting (to the information systems strategic objectives) in nature. The essence of the systems analysis should focus on the root of the problem, which is the need for information. Only then should supplemental discussion concentrate on the computer-related issues, i.e., the type of software and the specific hardware that is needed.

The need for the right information

Technology, in itself, cannot provide all of the solutions to the problems identified in the healthcare system. In fact, the development of separate "silos" of information systems represents a significant barrier to integrating information systems and achieving centralized databases. However, the acceptance of the role of information systems and technology as an integral component of a decentralized model, delivering a seamless continuum of care, must be recognized. To this end, I promote a research protocol containing nine milestones:

1. Illustrate that getting patient access to better data and information, i.e., their Electronic Patient Record (EPR) leads to an improvement in health outcomes.
2. Illustrate that getting patients (or other stakeholders) to participate in the design process improves the health record (or system being designed).
3. Create and/or identify more meaningful metrics that can be used to illustrate the improvement in health outcomes and benefits that the EPR can make.
4. Research the value of information systems, and technology in general, in improving outcomes.
5. Research best way that technology should be designed and implemented to ensure effective networking of health data and information.
6. Work with patients to design a better EPR and decision support tool.
7. Implement the EPR, new IS and measure the improvement using the new metrics.
8. Illustrate that the better, and more enriched, the data are within an EPR, the better the health outcomes.

9. Extend the research results into practice gradually yet persistently!

Healthcare providers need to know where value is added for the patient in order to improve that value, and they need to be able to measure future improvements against what they are currently doing in order to know whether improvement has been achieved. Effective information systems and technology are necessary conditions for measuring and managing this improvement in quality. Our first treatment must be to recognize that information technology is a critical component for the continuation of the current healthcare system. This will not be easily accomplished.

Improve-IT (Indices to Measure Performance Relating Outcomes, Value and Expenditure from Information Technology)

There is very little evidence throughout all of healthcare that provides support to the hypothesis that better information will result in better health outcomes. This research institute, Improve-IT (www.improve-it-institute.org), is intended to create such a body of evidence.

Consider the case of a 68-year-old man who presents himself to the hospital with slightly worsening shortness of breath, cough and a history of congestive heart failure (CHF). Routine blood work as well as an x-ray of his chest is ordered. The x-ray shows moderate enlargement of the heart that was worse than previous, but no comparison could be made because the health records department is unable to find the previous x-ray (or the report) that was performed three months ago. Further, the blood work is returned from the lab during a nursing change of shift and goes overlooked. His results showed a serum potassium of 3.1 meq/l and a sodium of 127 meq/l, down from 3.9 and 137 respectively. Finally, his weight is up by 5 pounds since his last visit, but once again his previous lab test results and weight were not immediately available. The ER doctor makes a slight adjustment to his medications, suggests he see his primary care physician in a week, and sends him home. Two days later he collapses at the grocery store and is taken by ambulance to the emergency room where yet another chest x-ray and blood work-up is performed and he is admitted directly to the Intensive Care Unit (ICU).

From the above scenario, it's quite evident that information technology (IT) can play a large and direct role in improving healthcare delivery. This is not an isolated case; every day many such cases exist where everyone would benefit from improved IS and IT. Then why have we not seen the evidence in the literature? Why is there no (or at least, very little) research showing this type of relationship – spending on IT leads to greater system availability which leads to increased clinician use which leads to improved decision-making which leads to improved health outcomes?

The answer is quite simple: We have not been very good at tracking IS and IT spending, system availability and utilization, and we do not measure health outcomes well!

Improve-IT is a research project that is intended to address these issues and to ultimately demonstrate the relationship between information management technology and better health outcomes. Further, we wish to show not only that there are benefits from IT investment, but also that the timing of these benefits, as well as the critical success factors, may vary.

In essence, we believe that there are three categories of measures that must be created. These are:

1. an accurate measure of total IT spending throughout the hospital
2. a detailed measure of the infusion of IT in the organization (where infusion is defined as both the scope and the timing of implementation and adoption)
3. an array of health outcomes comprised of a small number of existing performance indicators that can be linked to IT and objectively, and easily, calculated.

To accomplish this, we are creating a collaborative research network that will define specific measurement indicators, measure these indicators across organizations and publish results that will illustrate not only the existence, but also the timing, of health outcome benefits derived from ICT investment.

Subsequently, Improve-IT research network members, and eventually representatives from any interested healthcare institution, will be required to enter data that defines their organization and its IS capabilities, use, cost, and effectiveness. They will then be able to review and track their institution's performance over time against all the other sites, which will not be specifically identified, and a set of National and International benchmarks. In the end, healthcare system management (either in government, at a state or provincial level, or in delivering care, as in HMOs or large regional integrated systems) will be provided the necessary decision support facts and details so as to manage it with improved efficiency and effectiveness.

Prescription Two
Develop a National Patient Advocacy Program (NPAP)

The second prescription is to create this National Patient Advocacy Program, described earlier. This Program would not only have the capacity to continue doing the type of research and analysis needed, but would also be involved in educating patients and providing individuals the skills necessary to manage their health and consequently, the healthcare delivery more effectively.

We must begin to focus the discussion on what our healthcare system will look like in the future rather than lament over the past. The main premise of improved information systems is that incorporating a collaborative attitude toward information management throughout the community could affect increased efficiencies and improve quality of care.

So how do we get there? We all know that this will not be easy because if it were, we would have done it by now! One thing is certain: My saying that it needs to happen, or individual consumers fighting through individual battles, will not get it done either. This must be organized, coordinated and financed. In this way, we will be represented by a group that will have influence in the future design of our healthcare system. This is due to the fact that it will officially represent the entire patient perspective – comprised of the sick as well as the healthy public.

Studying the patient-doctor relationship
It's time for patients to demand improved information systems. Firstly, even though it is the law under freedom of information, it is very difficult to get access to one's own medical record, at

least in full. Secondly, information concerning performance of hospitals (for example) regarding financial position or mortality rates is next to impossible to ascertain. Thirdly, a full listing of physicians and their areas of specialty and corresponding performance in each area is not readily available. These types of information are not available for many reasons, but mainly because they do not exist, anywhere. One may argue that a medical chart exists – and this is correct. However, a full and comprehensive medical record that integrates information, which can be disseminated efficiently (i.e., electronically) across all healthcare providers, still, today, does not exist anywhere in the world.

All of the players in our healthcare system (doctors, nurses, clinicians, hospitals, providers) have a significant contribution to make, however, ultimately, it is the patient that must take responsibility for his/her own healthcare. The public must, individually and collectively, educate itself about health options and demand to be educated when the information is not forthcoming.

But what do the patient stakeholders want? Unfortunately, the patients have not been able to get their voice heard. This is, in part, due to a lack of organization. More importantly, there has been a lack of communication between the other health stakeholders and the patients regarding the need for the patients to contribute their information needs into the developmental process.

As a result of all of these factors, we must now create a National Patient Advocacy Program both in Canada and the United States. It is my objective to coordinate the genesis of this NPAP through the Improve-IT Institute described in Prescription One. It is planned that the profits from the sale of this book will go directly toward the creation and to the continued funding of this Program. Some of the functions of the NPAP are to:

1. Lobby and negotiate the patient interest at all health industry meetings
2. Support individual groups trying to affect change in healthcare
3. Support individual patients seeking ways to improve either the management of their care or the management of their information
4. Support all of the membership regarding patient education initiatives.

It is imperative that the patient stakeholder group becomes active and effective within the management of the healthcare system as soon as possible. Ideally, this should be a government-funded organization with a national focus. Once again, we can borrow a model from another industry. In October 2001, the Financial Consumer Agency of Canada (FCAC) was created to oversee consumer protection measures in the federally regulated financial services sector and to expand consumer education activities. Between June and October 2002, more than 3,600 consumers contacted the FCAC to lodge complaints and seek clarification on a variety of topics. This total number is comprised of consumers contacting the FCAC through its Consumer Contact Centre, their Web site, email and regular mail. Surely, if we can do this for the financial services, we must be able to see the benefit in health services!

Years ago, before television, people listened to radio for a portion of their evening's entertainment and one of the hits of the time was Jack Benny's Sunday evening show which was performed live. For one episode of the show, during rehearsal or so the story goes, they came upon a scene where Jack's character gets robbed by a man holding a gun. The robber asks: "Your money or your life?" Jack was not happy with the answer originally written into the script so they tried for a while during rehearsal to come up with something better... but could not. However, like the true professional he was, Jack stated that his creative genius would come alive during the performance and he would come up with something better during the show.

Sure enough, during the live show on Sunday night they got to the part where the robber asks, "Your money or your life?" Unfortunately, Jack was stumped and there was a pause on the air. So the actor playing the robber, taking a cue from acting school, buys Jack a little more time and repeats the line: "Your money or your life?" Jack, feeling the pressure, finally exclaimed: "I'm thinking it over!" Even though that was more a response to his fellow actor, his genius had indeed kicked in and created a classic Jack Benny line, which has been repeated many times since.

When it comes to what's important in our society today, for some reason we seem to have missed the joke and have emphasized the management of our money more than the management of our life (or health). Interesting point to consider.

Looking at my own experience, it was approximately ten years ago that my mother was diagnosed with breast cancer. My mother turned to me for advice because of my fluency with the healthcare industry. But where does the average patient go to get information about health services in the community? Where do we go to get a second opinion? How do I find out what hospitals are best at certain procedures? Who is the best doctor to perform this surgery?

Unfortunately, we do not, at present, have the data or information to properly answer any of these questions in an objective and systematic manner. Consequently, the Improve-IT Institute (www.improve-it-institute.org) must also develop healthcare evaluation metrics for use by patients to support the management of their own or a family member's personal care on an individual basis. Integrating system performance measures with health outcomes will allow for economies of scale (regarding the supporting infrastructure) and additional synergies (with respect to education and assistance).

Prescription Three
Begin the process of patient education

To date, all of my research has focused on one concept – better information in the right and most accessible format will improve decision-making. A research effort into defining the right information and the most accessible is required as these issues cannot be resolved through intuition alone, as we have seen throughout all of the stories that I have relayed. This research effort, however, cannot begin without first creating a data model and information systems within which analysis and innovation can take place. Once this living laboratory has been developed, different information structures can be tested and performance measured. Only through this research can the twofold education process begin: patients educating the health system about what they want and the system educating patients about what is possible and how patients can exercise their own health management.

Training and education play a significant role in the development of patient information systems as well because most patients do not have a sense of what comprises their health record let alone the value of the information contained therein. Consequently, if we advocate that patients must be more proactive in their health management and we propose that they access an information system containing their EPR, then it is a straightforward argument that the patients must be educated around technology and healthcare records.

This education and support initiative is the key as it interacts directly with the perceptions and expectations of all the constituents, patients and clinicians, regarding communication of new ideas and the ability to effect change in the organization. For example, one significant hurdle to overcome is to convince patients and healthcare providers to allow the very electronic transfer of their medical and patient information that is at the core of a new eHealth-based (or electronic delivery of health services) delivery system.

We're making the assumption that it's useful to understand and amplify the factors that influence decision making and that this understanding will enable better decision making in the future. The physician-patient group is distinct as it concerns decision-making reflecting both the individual and the population level. Hopefully, the patient will soon be seen to be an active decision maker in the healthcare field.

It is my belief that we must develop Internet-based educational material that can then be applied to help overcome the presence of doctor-patient, professional-cultural impediments to effective communication and decision-making.

To date, we have seen the patients demand:

- The volume and rate of specific causes (diseases) and purposes (procedures) of hospitalization
- Resources where they could go with respect to their own diagnosis
- The number of physicians and hospitals providing care for specific causes and purposes
- The number and type of high technology diagnostic tests and treatments used by residents of a particular community
- Healthcare expenditure on hospital care, ambulatory care, and other types of healthcare
- The number and location of primary care physicians with open practices
- Patient satisfaction data from previous/existing patients
- Measures of community integration across the healthcare system (i.e., networking the EPR)
- Special programs available at hospitals, group practices, and other healthcare institutions for community members.

Recent research

One good example of innovative research in practice is the recent work that I have been involved with in developing an interface for patients to access their own health record within a safe environment. This research is cutting edge in the world as we are exploring both patient and physician preferences regarding in-hospital and discharge information. As we move ahead, we are examining not only what information patients want but also how and when they want it. We are also focusing on physician preferences for both attending (in-hospital) and family doctors.

As an outcome of recent patient and physician preference research, the following insights were provided. Attending physicians and residents felt that patients should have access to self-care instructions, medication regimens and future appointments. However, less than half felt that the patient access should include hospital discharge summaries, and fewer than 20 percent agreed with inclusion of results of laboratory, ECG and radiographic examinations as well as operative reports. Nearly 60% of attending physicians and 80% of trainees felt that patients do not follow self-care instructions correctly post-discharge and access to the EPR could improve this statistic. Two of the attending physicians cited the potential for patient misinterpretation of data, particularly if the wording of reports included such terms as "borderline," and felt that patients may demand further investigation when it may not be medically necessary.

In contrast, nearly 100% of community-based family physicians felt that patients should have access to all documentation contained in the EPR, and that the patient access should integrate illness-specific information to further patient self-education. Sixty percent of family physicians reported that most patients do not follow self-care correctly post-discharge, and felt that patient access to an EPR would improve this statistic.

Clearly, there is going to be some element of resistance to change that will emanate from the physician group. Not all doctors will embrace change for all of the reasons we have enumerated for every other group. However, as students are similar in roles to patients, so too are the professors at a University very much like doctors. When we first introduced the DET (Chapter 5, the Education story), the faculty members were not enamored with our ideas either. A couple of early adopters saw the benefit and plunged ahead. Unfortunately, these leaders exhibited tremendous growing pains to the point that their course preparation time went up by an order of magnitude (i.e., almost ten times as long). When this word spread, there were not too many professors lining up to volunteer. However, over time the students began forcing many of the teachers to move ahead because they got to see the functionality and improvement in outcomes. This was a great illustration of how the consumerism (exhibited by students) took the change forward through the mere size in numbers of their group. It is my opinion that the patients group, at the right time, will begin to drive the change in healthcare to the point that the physicians will just have to get on board.

Ten of the 15 patient participants surveyed wanted access to the entire content of the EPR. All of these ten patients also identified themselves as technologically literate, whereas the five remaining patients self-identified as technologically illiterate. However, all patients, regardless of this self-assessment, unanimously wanted the EPR to include detailed supporting information on medications, including explanation of their purpose, drug interaction warnings, and a detailed description of side effects. Ninety percent of patients wanted inclusion information about the potential course of their illness in their electronic personal health record.

Further, 60% of patients felt that having access to their medical records would be helpful in self-management at home, and that this access would improve self-understanding of their medical condition, although 40% also believed that there would be no difference in their overall health (i.e., health outcomes) with this access. Sixty percent felt that both they and their physician would be the primary users of the electronic record access.

Despite self-reported computer literacy (70% reported beginner or moderate level of computer knowledge) among these patients, over 60% would also prefer receiving a summary of their record in paper format.

In our pilot survey, patients wanted to have access to all their information, and family physicians agreed that access to their complete record is beneficial. Physicians in the hospital saw less benefit and more potential danger in this access. This lack of consensus between community-based and hospital-based physicians may be related to the nature of the physician-patient relationship that subsequently develops. In the hospital, a more paternalistic relationship construct may be a matter of necessity because the presence of an urgent medical situation and patients may be less able or less interested in participation in decision making. In the community, patients are less acutely ill and more active participants in their care. The type of relationship that naturally develops between themselves and their physicians may be more conducive to greater patient autonomy.

Future studies of chronic patients may also eventually yield disease-specific EPR usage patterns, drawing into question the validity of studies in which patients with different illness care plans and self-management issues are grouped together. Chronically ill patients have indicated that both they and their physicians should have equal utilization of an electronic record, and this may be reflective of how the disease management program is constructed. Home-based self-management programs for diabetes, for example, in which a patient has daily responsibility to self-test, may have greater use, and hence measurably greater benefit from having access to their records.

The impact of health information and data provision does not end when the patient leaves the physician's office or shuts down the computer. This may explain why computer literate patients would also want supplemental paper copies of their hospital records. Family members often assist patients at home as they try to convert complex information from paper or electronic records into usable knowledge. Anxiety reduction and other benefits from any information intervention may be maximized if a patient is able to discuss the information with those whom they trust. This is particularly relevant when measuring outcomes from the implementation of remote access to electronic records because patients could potentially view their records twenty-four hours a day with whomever they choose. This also limits the generalizability of findings from patients observed in usability laboratories to real-life Web-based EPR access.

Finally, patient-centred implementation of any information system occurs within the context of an existing healthcare organization. The divergent opinions between physicians and patients in our pilot study about the appropriate extent of patient access underscore the need for a realistic organizational assessment of the willingness of medical staff and administration to support the type of cultural shift that accompanies this democratized access to previously protected archives.

Informatics advancements such as patient access to an EPR transform the patient from a passive recipient of care to an active participant in clinical decision making, augmenting patient self-efficacy and knowledge creation, and that can lead to an improvement in health outcomes. However, if there is inadequate leadership and vision to counter substantial resistance to this cultural shift, then the realized return on investment for any technology promoting further patient empowerment, whether measured in terms of fiscal, health or clinical outcomes, may be minimal. In the end, communication of expectations is the cornerstone of successful information technology adoption.

During my doctoral studies, I came across the theory of Know-Don't Know. In essence, everything in our lives is split into three groups:

1. what people *know they know*;
2. what people *know they don't know*; and
3. what people *don't know they don't know*.

For clarification, we can define these categories simply with examples. First, you know, for example, where you live, your children's names and your job (at least, for the most part!). Second, you know nuclear physics, as a discipline, exists even though you may not know any of the details. Finally, you didn't know anything about Kevin Leonard before reading this book (maybe that's a bad example because you may now wish you'd stayed ignorant) and so you didn't know that you didn't know!

The unfortunate thing is that many believe that we need to expand the first area – learn the details about everything. Albert Einstein said it best when he stated that we do not need to know everything, we just need to know where everything is to basically reduce the third area and expand area number two. It is not our job as patients to learn the entire health system or go to medical school; but we do need to know more about our personal and health delivery system options and to find out who has the most knowledge in specific areas when we need assistance or care. This is very much like when we manage our finances – we don't know every tax rule but we do know how to find the phone number for a tax specialist. Right now, there is no such support mechanism that can help individual patients navigate the system more effectively. In addition, overall system performance evaluation from a multitude of perspectives is severely lacking. Therefore, a program of advocacy, such as I am proposing here as the NPAP, is needed to fill this gap in service and support. Herein, we will continue to conduct research projects examining the types of data and information that will empower the patient most effectively. (Updates to research and recent findings will be available at the Improve-IT web site: www.improve-it-institute.org.)

Consequently, I ask you to join me along a journey of learning and innovation. There is enough work for all of us. Remember, we don't have to try to do or know everything. Our goal should be to expand just that part of the KNOW/ DON'T KNOW area so that the information is there when and if we need it. The more we accomplish, the more we will attract new people to new ideas and philosophies and expand current, and often very limiting, boundaries.

Prescription Four
*Begin the public debate about the specific issues
relating to healthcare services*

The final prescription involves the need to determine the characteristics of a health system that the public wants: in other words, answers to questions like "What are the good things about the way things work today?" More importantly, what are the things that do not work and require improvement? The idea is to acknowledge that patients should participate not only in the management of their own care but also in the change that is needed at the system level. If not, then a very powerful and contributing force will be left on the outside of the system looking in ... *again.*

In order to accomplish this, we need to get together in public forums and have a debate about the pros and cons of our healthcare system. The creation of the NPAP provides a natural forum for the genesis of these debates. Below, I present some of the areas and questions that require discussion and solutions. (*These issues can also be found on the Improve-IT web site, www.improve-it-institute.org, where anyone can get involved in the "virtual public debate" by posting messages and ideas on the electronic bulletin boards.*)

Herein, I do not provide a speculative response or even a recommendation as I believe these decisions should only be made after much debate and only then by a collective health industry stakeholder entity which would be comprised of doctors, hospital representatives, other groups and patients. These four broad categories are:

I. STRATEGIC

What is our Vision for the health system going forward?
This is, by far, the biggest issue that is facing our healthcare system today. We need to very quickly decide what the structure of the delivery system should be and how we should manage it. In addition, we must set a course for the infusion of electronic media into and throughout the system. For example, there are those who believe that to get the type of benefits that other industries have garnered from technology, we need to go toward the path of one patient – one record. Others argue that that would be too costly and we should orient ourselves to the concept of a read-only, browser-based, virtual comprehensive EPR. Others still want something somewhere in the middle between these two extremes. In addition, we need to discuss the feasibility of the creation of a HealthBank and what role this plays in the management of the future of health delivery.

Are we happy with the system we have now or should we investigate ways to bring in more private sector participation?
As explained in an earlier discussion, there is a difference between the concept of a "two-tiered" system and private sector involvement. That being said, there still needs to be input from the different stakeholder groups around for-profit business contributing and/or managing health delivery organizations.

Where do we stand with respect to the need to protect privacy and confidentiality versus the substantial gains from effective computer integration?
We must determine what level of protection is acceptable to

the public. This is very difficult to identify in the abstract, thus much work will need to be done to prepare for this discussion. Further, we must determine the level of appropriate compensation for individuals when their privacy has been breached (see 7 below for more discussion).

Are we willing to fiscally trade off some of our other social programs in order to save healthcare?

Another area that has been raised in the past, albeit infrequently, is the opportunity to put more money into the healthcare system by borrowing, perhaps on a short-term basis only, from other social programs. Once again, the discussion around this topic will be hotly contested and will require a large degree of commitment on behalf on the politicians to stick it through.

In a recent development, the state of Tennessee has passed legislation that will limit patients' usage of the public healthcare system. As an example, all patients will have a cap on how many doctor visits and how many prescriptions will be funded. After the cap, patients (even those chronically ill) will then have to pay for services themselves! That legislation was passed without a consensus panel that should have included coordinated patient representation. After all, is it not the patients that fund the government in the first place through taxation? Perhaps we're prepared to make trade-offs to save healthcare, but we'll never know unless we have the debates.

II. TACTICAL

What are the issues surrounding a Universal Patient Identifier?

I've stated many times throughout this book that there is the need for a UPI and why it is important. What I have not discussed is how this type of identifier should be created and to what other areas it should be linked. Some provinces and HMOs have made great strides in this area, both in the acceptance of the concept and in moving forward with implementation. However, many questions remain unanswered: Should we have a common UPI infrastructure across all of the country? Should this UPI link us to other government agencies? Obviously, further debate in these areas is required to determine the best possible solutions.

How do we start demonstrating the Business Case for IT?

Over the course of the debates and town hall meetings that must take place, the question of whether investment in information technology (or perhaps, more broadly, computers) is cost effective will have to be addressed. As stated, this will be very difficult to prove because the benefits and the costs can not be compared directly due to the fact that they are different measures: one is strictly in terms of dollars and time, while the other is comprised of health outcomes such as length of hospital stays, mortality, and other related metrics. Is saving one life from an adverse event (getting the wrong drug that may have killed the patient) worth $100,000? Or is it worth two lives? Where is the break-even point? How can one possibly answer these absurd questions and yet retain the integrity of the health system? It will be difficult and the solution may only appear over time, however these questions must be discussed and we must hear from the patient perspective.

III. OPERATIONAL

What shall we do when there is a breach of security?

As soon as the movement to EPRs has started in earnest, and to a large degree, it already has, we know, not propose, but know, there will be breaches to the system. Every computer system has had hackers and others attempt to log into their architecture and databases for financial gain, to wreak havoc or just because it is there. We cannot spend the next 100 years attempting to build the only IS in the world that will never have an attempt or breach to its security (which can also come in the form of employees inadvertently compromising the system).

It's worth noting that any electronic record keeping will be at less risk and have fewer breaches than the system employed today – a point that often goes unmentioned by those in the resistance-to-change camp. The cases of records being faxed to wrong fax numbers, health records being sold (unwittingly, of course) while remaining in old filing cabinets and even clinicians losing files while making home care ,calls, are too numerous to document. Needless to say, security is not running at 100% efficiency today. It's just that very few people are aware of this fact due to the limited nature of the number of people involved. In other words, the fear with EPRs is that the data breached can be distributed widely in a short matter of time. Therefore, we need some mechanism to audit the new e-health systems and a process for providing retribution or compensation for those that then suffer from the consequence.

How do we build a system with an effective balance between accountability and responsibility?

There is a need for consistent performance measures all across this industry. These measures will rate doctor or health provider effectiveness. How do we get the contribution from the clinicians? Where do we publish the results? Is it reasonable to expect an objective measure of performance rating? Clearly, there must be both responsibility and accountability. One cannot impose outcome measures and then not have them mean anything or have no one there with the responsibility to improve performance or to make sure the measurement is ongoing! If we are going to improve the health system, then measurement is a must! The question is how and who should be responsible? This could be performed by a patient advocacy group either alone or in partnership with other health stakeholders.

What comprises an emergency health record? Is this the same as a Health Data Packet described earlier?

This feature was presented in Chapter 7 in conjunction with a proposed Health Vision statement and the need to exchange data within an electronic health record in an effort to create a virtual EPR. Representation from all stakeholders must be present to identify the details of this concept in its entirety.

IV. ONGOING

How do we ensure that the system we design today stays in place and continues to grow with our needs as a country?

No matter how much planning and forethought there is, there will always be events or circumstances that just cannot be forecasted that will affect the whole system. If there was any doubt before about this fact, there should not be any now after the SARS – Severe Acute Respiratory Syndrome – outbreak in Toronto in early 2003. We must build an infrastructure that is resilient to such events, one that will not meet a catastrophic end when something unforeseen arises. This means that a National Patient Advocacy Programme must be supported and an infrastructure put in place that is robust.

INVOLVEMENT IN SYSTEM DESIGN

As can easily be seen, there are a number of complex issues that have not yet been resolved and have no straightforward, obvious best solution. Consequently, the need for a public debate is evident more now than at any other time in our history.

In the recent academic literature, it is becoming increasingly recognized that collaboration between different professional-cultural groups is a critical component of the movement to achieve consistent quality in patient care and improved overall institutional performance. This is now especially important as new information systems are making data and good quality evidence more and more available to all parties.

Consequently, there exists a tremendous need to address the barriers of effective decision making between groups which are separated either in the same or in different organizations and/or in distance within the same or between different disciplines. These barriers depend on many factors including the previous training of the individuals and the basic tenets such as commonality of terms. Researchers must focus on the patient perspective, i.e., the needs of the patient; the changes in healthcare that are long overdue; the inpatient versus home care debate. Finally, we need to examine patients' personal healthcare lifestyle objectives and information needs. Only through public input and debate can we arrive at creative solutions that satisfy objectives from a multi-stakeholder perspective.

As an example, a recent article in the newspaper *USA Today* (Thursday July 1, 2004; story on Steve Woodle) described a saving of a life event through patient active involvement and decision-making. In fact, the patient was credited by his doctors for acting fast and not waiting for his condition to worsen. In this particular case, however, the patient himself was a physician. Obviously, the health system is more accepting of this patient's involvement because of his credentials. I think this is also a great illustration of the bigger issue of how technology and patient managed care can work within our healthcare systems to produce improved outcomes. The patient/doctor was quoted as saying that "becoming a patient has made him a better doctor." Hopefully, all patients will not have to become doctors to get input into their care!

One final story

After graduation from my doctoral studies, I wanted to take a break from academia and try my hand at the real world. As my dissertation was in the area of banking and credit, I was interested in working in the financial sector and ended up getting a job in the Securities department of the Bank of Canada in Ottawa. One of my first tasks was to produce the Briefing Notes (from our department) for the Governor of the Bank in time for the regular Board of Directors meetings that were held every six weeks or so. After watching my predecessor do the task for one six-week cycle, I was handed the job and was assured that if I had any questions she would be available. However, everything seemed very straightforward – even simplistic – why would I need to contact her?

Over the next six weeks, I set about gathering data and producing information like nobody's business. I created new charts, coloured graphs, changed legends and even re-ordered the reports so substantially that there was hardly anything resembling the old Briefing Notes in my new and improved format. In my opinion, this was much more structured and the data was now being represented in such a way so as to provide vivid information on trends and events.

Needless to say, that was the only time I prepared the Briefing Notes. I know what you're thinking – he did such a great job he was promoted to Deputy Governor on the spot! Not quite. It appears that no one else thought they resembled the old Briefing Notes either, and that was the problem. They didn't want a new format or an elaborate reconstruction, at least, not without their input. What I did was go ahead and rebuild the system (as a system designer) without the contribution of the users and stakeholders involved – a perfect recipe for failure. The rest of my tenure at the Bank, I'm happy to say, contained nowhere near the same amount of drama; I later moved to the consulting sector of financial services in the United States.

We, as patients, *must* be involved in the system design changes for the future if we are to play a larger stakeholder role therein.

CHAPTER NINE

Final Remarks

To paraphrase Ralph Waldo Emerson: "We have not inherited the healthcare system from our fathers, but rather we are borrowing it from our children."

We have been patient long enough! Now that we know the issues facing healthcare and what some of the short-term treatments must be, where do we go from here?

Over the last number of years, we have been inundated with government and private industry studies on what ails the healthcare system and what is needed. The primary solution always presented is money: "We recommend that we allocate a budget of x billion dollars so we can _____ (fill in the blank)." After this point, the studies begin to differ depending on the scope and the direction of the mandate of the research. Some studies have focused on emergency room over-crowding, wait-lists for surgery or home care. There have even been studies that have recommended that more money should be invested into information technology. In short, these studies recommend changes or advancements in their specific areas or for the whole healthcare system (as in the case of the Romanow Commission, 2002).

After the investment recommendation, however, there is little detailed guidance as to how to improve the healthcare system. This is a consistent theme because the problems are complex and the solutions are not obvious. We do know one thing, however, and that is that talking about the problems and stating that we must find a way to do something has not been helpful.

WHAT ARE THE TAKEAWAYS FROM THIS BOOK?

While it is true that there are no definite solutions articulated herein, I have presented an outline in terms of objectives and next steps describing the progression from where we are today to where we need to be. These are summarized below. The main emphasis is that the patient stakeholder group must be active in the healthcare revolution that is taking place. Once that becomes evident, the discussion among all stakeholders will be more effective as the users/payers of the system will finally be involved in the process.

Let's review the issues one final time:

- There is very poor overall management information
- There are inadequate information systems
- There is fragmentation of information and healthcare delivery
- There is inadequate accountability and measurement
- There is inefficient electronic connectivity between institutional and community care
- There is heterogeneous data recording, lack of a standardized terminology, lack of system linking and ineffective access to stored information

- There is massive resistance to change across many stakeholder groups
- There is a lack of technology-use sophistication
- There is poor performance measures and outcome evaluation
- There is a lack of competition anywhere in the delivery system (e.g., hospitals, doctors, clinics) that would otherwise drive technology use through the need for all to retain or obtain competitive advantage.

Consequently, we need:

- better health information in all areas of healthcare
- a virtual centralized patient data registry containing some degree of electronic patient record
- to overcome ignorance concerning computers and IS
- to overcome resistance to change
- to educate patients regarding the role of IT and around the value of their health information (provide access and demonstrate the contents of their EPR)
- to develop integrated information and integrated delivery systems
- to address privacy and confidentiality concerns within a computerized health world
- ultimately, in order to accomplish all of the above, a National program to support patients in both the decision making and the execution of those decisions!

Generally speaking, we will need to re-orient ourselves from a system that is institutionally founded to one where the patient is truly at the centre. Some of this shift will comprise the following:

Focus of current information systems
- Institutional patient identifier
- Information access only within 4 walls
- Information capture after care is delivered
- No sharing of data with other providers
- Single provider clinical pathways
- Based on single episode of care
- Acute illness
- Institutional cost, quality, outcome data
- Patient data.

Focus of future information systems
- System patient ID – unique patient identifier (UPI)
- Information retrieval from anywhere in the system
- Information capture as care is delivered
- Sharing of data with other system providers
- Multi-provider clinical pathways
- Customer/member service
- Wellness and prevention of hospitalization
- System cost, quality, outcome data
- Patient and population demographic and health status data.

The concept of a unique patient identifier (UPI) across the entire health system is a necessary condition for any truly integrated and improved health system, as it will allow the providers to access a patient's health record regardless of where the patient appears in the continuum of care. Once accessed, clinical information is entered in the record as care is delivered which ensures that the record is always current. The fact that providers share an information system means that a provider can review the care that the patient has received from other healthcare providers, eliminating duplicate tests, histories, and so on.

Clinical pathways that transcend providers optimizes the care and ensures that patients receive the right care at the right time – the focus is on what is happening to the patient in total and not just a single episode of care. Clinicians and care managers will use the system cost, quality, and outcome information to improve basic processes of care. New clinical information will be used to develop strategies to prevent further disease and re-hospitalization. Patients will be able to more effectively handle day-to-day living by staying on top of their most recent health indicators (e.g., blood sugar level, blood pressure). Information about population health status is used for the ongoing process of health planning and evaluation.

To date, there has been much fear mongering from within the healthcare system by those who are the most ardent resistors to change. These individuals and organizations state unequivocally that patients' biggest fear is security (what happens if there is a breach of security?), referencing research studies or just stating their gut intuition. Is this true? Are patients so fearful that we have put off the technology revolution in healthcare? With information being in electronic format, the argument is that not only can a breach happen, the magnitude can potentially be very large. The bottom line is that, to date, there has been no such debate or research. In fact, that is one of the major objectives of this book, to find out what patients want. How can we know what the patient public wants before we ask them?

On the contrary, it is my belief that patients want to be progressive and move ahead. We all have more confidence in technology than say, 15 years ago. As a result, patients in general will support the movement to electronic healthcare. There is no way of knowing with certainty unless this group is canvassed. A National Patient Advocacy Program (NPAP) is the best opportunity to get represented and involved so as to get the patient voice heard. (*For more information, contact www.improve-it-institute.org.*) In the end, it truly is that simple! We must begin today.

You may ask: "Why should we believe that there is a need to create a National Patient Advocacy Programme? Why should we believe this author? I have attempted to outline my credibility by documenting my experience, which in turn provides a framework for my current perspective of Canada's and, to some extent, the United States' health delivery systems. In the end, however, someone has to begin this journey and I ask you to help me advance this industry together. Eventually, the most effective management and leadership will emerge. In the interim, however, who better to lead the charge to save our healthcare system than someone who the healthcare system has already saved many times? As a result of what it has done for me, I am very passionate about improving healthcare. I also believe that passion defines skill. In other words, the people who have the passion for a task will always do it best; give the job to someone who wants to do it.

Can patient empowerment truly save our healthcare system? I firmly believe it can due to the current use of the health services. In a recent US study, the results indicate that more than 70% of all healthcare costs are spent on chronically ill patients, a group which makes up less than 20% of the population! If we provide information to these high users of the system and these few become more effective in improving their health outcomes, the cost savings alone can prove to be very large indeed.

We must continue to fight for the long-term decision over short-term gains; this will require adopting the concept of working smarter (with higher short-term costs) and letting go of the old philosophy of working harder, which only works in the very short run. In the end, the technology curve illustrates that a total effort reduction is the reward in the long term (after Time 4). It takes tremendous courage to stop bailing (working harder) when the ship is sinking and take time to find the hole (working smarter) but ultimately, that is the only way to save the crew.

> It must be re-emphasized that the alternatives presented in this book are discussed so as to provide a platform or starting point for further debate. I am not espousing any single architectural design to the information systems but rather that we need improved IS and, as patients, this cannot happen without our involvement. The best, final solution can only be determined with the public input.

As we progress, we will hit many roadblocks, many of which have been discussed here. For example, patients may find it, at least at the outset, very disturbing to examine the intimate details of their own file (or health record). They may find that it takes more work than it used to when their physician did all the homework. The success rate of new systems could fall prey to the same problems as physician information systems, that is, being data rich and information poor. These challenges will arise. This is known and it will happen to some degree with certainty, therefore none of us should be surprised when it does. What we must do is support the move to improved IS through our collective involvement and commit to staying the

222 • KEVIN J. LEONARD

course and being the pioneers or early adopters that are very much needed at this time on our history.

In conclusion, I would like to leave you with one last story that I have borrowed from Stephen Denning (*The Springboard*, page 132).

— • —

"There was this old man who lived in a village and he was what you would call eccentric ... He was really quite wise ... gave people advice about how to start a business, or raise their crops or their children in such a way that he was never wrong, and so everybody tolerated his wackiness, and went to him for advice.

"Now there were two little boys in the village who decided to play a trick on him ... what they decided to do was capture a small bird, and then in the town square in front of everyone, they were going to confront the old man. One of the boys was going to hold the bird behind his back, and he was going to ask the old man what he had. And if the old man could guess, then he would ask him whether it was alive or dead. If the old man said it was dead, he would let it fly away in front of everyone and make a fool of him right there on the spot. Or if he said that it was alive, he would crush the bird and drop it at his feet, making a fool of him either way. That was the plan.

"So one day when the old man was at the town square and everyone was gathered around, the little boys set about hunting. Poor baby sparrow! They captured the bird and they went up to him. When everyone was in earshot, the biggest boy held the bird and the littlest boy said, 'What's my friend got behind his back?'

"The old man looked at him a long time. That was how he had become so wise. He looked until he saw a little sparrow's feather drifting down behind the boy's legs. 'Well it's a sparrow, isn't it? A baby sparrow.'

"Everyone's eyes grew wide. But the little boy piped up just as fast, 'Well is it alive? Or is it dead?'

"The old man looked at that boy, because he knew what he was really asking. And then he looked at the boy who was holding the bird. He looked at him until that boy looked back at him. 'Well,' he said, 'the answer to that is in your hands.'"

— • —

Clearly, the answer to all of the questions pertaining to the future of our healthcare system is indeed in our hands. We must decide whether we wish to be involved in this process or not. If we do not participate then we may not get the system that the majority of Canadians want. If we do, then we will play a defining role in the shape and scope of the system. There are many active and powerful stakeholder groups: hospitals, government, private industry (pharmaceuticals, technology firms) and clinicians. However, there is no group more powerful than the collective patient group – but we have yet to coordinate and get involved. We can make a difference. It's our choice. It is in our hands!

"Looks like we're stepping up to the challenge [of electronic health records]. And for once, Canadians might be the leader – in no small measure thanks to a public health system where the provinces are cooperating around a nationwide initiative."

David Ticoll,
author, speaker, consultant, *The Globe and Mail*,
Thursday, September 11, 2003

AFTERWORD

More than 100 years ago, Sir William Osler said: "Listen to the patient and the patient will give you the diagnosis." This engaging book represents a loud cry that asks for more involvement of patients in decisions about their health and health care. The author, Dr. Kevin Leonard, is someone who knows the health system very well and who has experienced it, at its best and worst, as a patient throughout most of his life. He also witnessed, both as an insider and as a customer, how the financial world changed, irreversibly, after the introduction of online transactions. Daunted by the wide gap between what the health system could be and what it is, Dr. Leonard has challenged us all to bring patients from the periphery of the health system to its core. The message is clear: Patients deserve respect and an opportunity to participate actively in decisions that could have profound effects on their health and health care. Will the health system listen to it? I hope it does.

At a time when most health systems around the world are struggling to meet increasing needs for health services with limited resources, we have an urgent need for innovation. A savvy and engaged public, coupled with powerful information and communication technologies (ICTs) might be the perfect recipe for an innovative burst.

With the rapidly declining costs of technology, electronic communication tools are booming. Simple text-based e-mail could be used by patients and health professionals to deal with time-consuming tasks that now require face-to-face consultations such as the description of normal laboratory test results, the renewal of prescriptions and the arrangement of appointments. Similarly, digital cameras could be used to capture images that sent through the Internet could be assessed at a distance, eliminating the need for unnecessary visits to specialists. Fast Internet access coupled with cheap Web cameras are already allowing live tele-consultations through telephones and personal computers. All of these possibilities, and the many others that we cannot anticipate now, could lead to more balanced and productive relationships between the public and health professionals, to the creation of new health services and patterns of work, and to efficient allocation of the resources available.

However, thinking that fancy gadgets alone will lead to a radically different health system, is naïve. Creating the humane, effective and efficient system that people deserve and expect will require unprecedented levels of generosity and collaboration among groups that have traditionally been self-centred and competitive. This book invites us all to meet the challenge. Let's hope we listen and act soon.

Alejandro (Alex) R. Jadad, MD DPhil FRCPC
Director, Centre for Global eHealth Innovation; Canada Research Chair in eHealth Innovation; Rose Family Chair in Supportive Care; Professor, Faculty of Medicine; University Health Network and University of Toronto; Toronto, Canada

When we received the detailed biography of Dr. Leonard, it took 23 pages to spell out his accomplishments! Even in its condensed form we required four pages of curriculum vitae. We feel, in bringing to the reader, it is important that they have an overview of the man who feels the importance of the topic is worth the time to bring his concerns to the public – the patients requiring healthcare in present and future years.

Dr. Kevin J. Leonard is a most unusual personality, known in North America and around the world for his advocacy on many issues, especially health and those of public concern.

Many of his lectures, seminars and speaking engagements will be built around the topics laid out so clearly in *A Prescription for Patience*, and we wish him well in his added career as a book author about topics of issue and public concern.

As publishers, we find Dr. Leonard to be a devoted author, accomplished to a fine degree in being able to present his views with clarity and determination.

White Knight is proud to add to its list of accomplished authors, this wonderful new talent.

Bill Belfontaine
Publisher

MORE ABOUT KEVIN J. LEONARD

CURRENT POSITIONS

Associate Professor,
      Department of Health Policy, Management and Evaluation
(HPME), Faculty of Medicine, University of Toronto, July
1996 - present.

Research Scientist,
      Centre for Global eHealth Innovation, University Health
Network (UHN), Toronto, Jan 2002 - present.

RECENT PUBLICATIONS:
PEER REVIEWED ACADEMIC JOURNALS:

Leonard, K.J., Lin, J., Dalziel, S., Yap, R. and Adams, D. (2004),
"Incorporating Operation Research Techniques to Evaluate
Information Systems Impact on Healthcare", <u>Journal of the
Operational Research Society (JORS)</u>, Volume 56, p. 173-
179.

Pederson, LT., and Leonard, K.J., (2005), "Measuring Information
Technology Investment Among Canadian Academic Health
Science Centres", <u>Electronic Healthcare,</u> Volume 3, Number
3, p. 94-101.

Leonard, K.J. (2004), "The Role of Patients in Designing Health
Information Systems: *The Case of Applying Simulation
Techniques to Design an Electronic Patient Record (EPR)
Interface*", <u>Health Care Management Science – Special Issue</u>,
Volume 7, Number 4, (November), p. 275-284.

Leonard, K.J. (2004), "Critical Success Factors Relating to Healthcare's
Adoption of New Technology: *A Guide to Increasing the
Likelihood of Successful Implementation*", <u>Healthcare Quarterly</u>,
Volume 7, Number 2, p. 72-81.

Winkelman, W.J., and Leonard, K.J. (2004), "Overcoming Structural
Constraints to Patient Utilization of Electronic Medical
Records: *A Critical Review and Proposal for an Evaluation
Framework*", <u>Journal of the American Medical Information
Association (JAMIA)</u>, Volume 11, Number 2, p. 151-161.

Leonard, K.J., Rauner, M., Schaffhauser-Linzatti, M.M., and Yap, R. (2002), "The Effect of Funding Policy on Day of the Week Admissions and Discharges in Hospitals: The cases of Austria and Canada", Health Policy, Volume 63 (3), p. 239-257.

Leonard, K.J. (2002), "The Use of Video Within a Database Management System: The creation of an integrated information system for National Hockey League (NHL) teams", International Journal of Computer Applications in Technology (IJCAT), Vol. 15, No. 6, p. 287-296.

Leonard, K.J., Wilson, D., and Malott, O. (2001), "Measures of Quality in Long Term Care Facilities", International Journal of Health Care Quality Assurance - Leadership in Health Services, Volume 14, Numbers 2 & 3, p.i-viii.

Leonard, K.J., and Smith, T. (2001), "A Faculty Perspective of the Adoption of On-Line Learning Technology in the MHSc Program at the University of Toronto: *Barriers and Enablers*", The Journal of Health Administration Education, Volume 19, Number 1 (Winter), p.89-99.

Leonard, K.J. (2000), "The Adoption of Distance Education Technology in a Master of Health Administration (MHA/MHSc) Curriculum: *Anecdotes and Antidotes*", The Journal of Health Administration Education, Volume 18, Number 3 (Summer), p. 321-333.

Leonard, K.J. (2000), "Information Systems for Healthcare: Why we have not had more success -*The Top 15 Reasons*", Healthcare Management Forum, Volume 13, Number 3 (Fall), p. 45-51.

SCHOLARLY ACTIVITIES

- Invited to send Credit Scoring Video and Manual to the National Library of Canada, 1993. Call number: HG3751.5L46; 1993 folio.

- Creation of Canadian Credit Risk Management Association (CCRMA) Elected Founding President, June 24, 1992.

- Graduation Ceremonies - Keynote Speaker

  "Credit and the Information Age", a speech given to the Credit Institute of Canada - Toronto Chapter, Nov 13, 1993.

- Software developed: Leonard, K.J., Pink, G.H., Richards, J.,

Leggat, S., Kelly, C., and Kelly, I., (1996-97) "Healthcare Interactive Simulation Exercise – HISE", HEALNet, Healthcare Management Theme.

- Directed two-year study of Grand River Hospital Departments (Kitchener-Waterloo Hospital site) to determine data flows and information needs. Supervised 30 MBA students per term over 4 terms. January 1995 to April 1996.

- Panellist for "A Vision for Health in Ontario: The Role of IT", Fair Share - televised by Rogers Community Cable 20, Public Forum on Health, sponsored the Mayors of Cambridge, Kitchener and Waterloo, Cambridge, Ontario, February 12, 1998.

Television Interviews
- CKCO, Six o'clock news hour interview, credit scoring and the retail industry, October, 1992.
- CKCO, Six o'clock news hour interview, CHIN Network, November 21,1996.
- CKCO, Six o'clock news hour interview, patient advocacy group, health industry, Feb. 12, 97.
- CITY-TV, Six o'clock news hour, patient advocacy issues, health industry, Nov 6, 1998.
- Discovery TV – Medical Hotseat Panellist – patient advocacy, rights to information, July 25, 04.

Radio Interviews
- 66CFR Calgary Flames Radio - Pre-game interview on the uses of computers in hockey, April, 1994.
- CBC Radio One – Describing play Coaching Matters, drive home with Avril Lavigne, Sept, 2002.

Newspaper Articles
- "Sharpening the tools for credit risk management", Laurier News, March 9, 1993, p. 3.
- "Laurier prof helps lenders cut their loan losses", Kitchener-Waterloo Record, Saturday, Apr. 10, 1993, p.B8.
- "Misplaced medical files delayed brain surgery", Kitchener-Waterloo Record, Monday, May 6, 1996, p.A1, Kitchener-Waterloo Record, Editorial, January, 1997.
- "The Need for Patient Awareness", Hamilton Spectator, November 15, 1998.

- "On With the Show, On With the Lecture", University of Toronto Bulletin, July 23, 2001, p.5.

— • —

In Addition:
- Received AWARD of Recognition for Community Service at CCAC Waterloo Annual Meeting - Sept 15 1999.
- Magazine/Newsletter Articles
  – "Decision Systems moves Risk Management Ahead", *The Information Source*, Volume VI, Number 3, Fall 1994, p.1.
  – "Advanced analytical skills help Kevin Leonard conquer new challenges", Commerce Today, Concordia University Newsletter, Volume 1, Number 4, Spring 1998, p. 6.
  – "What's the Score ... on Overrides", For SCORE Newsletter, CCRMA, Volume 7, Number 5, Summer, 1998, p. 1-2.
- 1988 Skit Row Winner for Best Skit Writing. Skit performed at National Arts Centre in Ottawa.
- Had my own original play, "Extensive Care", part of New Play Festival, Wilfrid Laurier University, April 25, 1993.
- Co-Founder and Executive Director of IMPROVE-IT Institute Institute to measure value of IT in healthcare; chaired first conference on failures, Toronto, November 11 and 12, 2004. IMPROVE-IT: Indices Measuring Performance Relating Outcomes, Value and Expenditure from Information Technology.

WHITE KNIGHT'S
"REMARKABLE WOMEN" SERIES

Conscious Women — Conscious Lives Book One

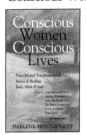

A book that lives up to expectations that women across North America constantly provide the nurturing component that continues to make our countries so great. These stories from across Canada and the United States of America, bring home those concern that women have for other women providing love, nourishment and hope for our present and future generations. Remarkable women, everyone. Thank you! ISBN 0-9734186-1-3 216 pages PB US $13.95 Cdn $19.95

Conscious Women — Conscious Lives Book Two

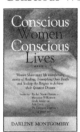

The second book in the Conscious Women — Conscious Lives series offers more extraordinary stories of healing and transformation by some of North America's leading women authorities on healing, spirituality and body, mind wisdom. Each story is true and each brings healing, understanding, comfort and proof of women's courage. ISBN 0-9736705-0-9 210 pages PB US $13.95 Cdn $19.95

Sharing MS

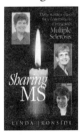

This informative book by the author and two women friends with Multiple Sclerosis, is a beacon of common sense lighting the way of those who have MS or suspect they may be afflicted, as well as being helpful to family, friends and health professionals. Read the book then call the MS Society Chapter in your local telephone book for information about your concerns regarding Multiple Sclerosis. ISBN 0-9730949-7-4 218 pages PB US $13.95 Cdn $19.95

The Unusual Life and Times of Nancy Ford-Inman

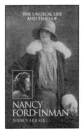

This story is about a most remarkable woman who contributed so much to Britain's literature, the theatre, media and the war effort in spite of a major physical handicap. Badly crippled by Cerebral Palsy at an early age yet she fought her way to become the author of almost 60 romantic novels and journalistic endeavors too numerous to count. ISBN 0-9730949-8-2 238 pages PB US $13.95 Cdn $19.95

To order, contact one of the distributors shown on the copyright page or be in touch with the book store nearest to you.

BOOKS BY
WHITE KNIGHT PUBLICATIONS

ADOPTION (Gay)
A Swim Against The Tide
    – David R.I. McKinstry

BIOGRAPHY
*The Life and Times of Nancy
Ford-Inman* – Nancy Erb Kee

HEALTH
Prescription for Patience
    – Dr. Kevin J Leonard

HUMOUR
*An Innkeeper's Discretion Book
    One & An Innkeeper's
    Discretion Book Two*
    – David R.I. McKinstry

INSPIRATION
*Conscious Women / Conscious
    Lives Book One
Conscious Women / Conscious
    Lives Book Two*
    – Darlene Montgomery
Happiness: Use It or Lose It
    – Rev. Dr. David "Doc"
    Loomis
*How I Became Father to
    1000 Children*
    – Rev. Dr. John S Niles
Sharing MS (Multiple Sclerosis)
    – Linda Ironside
Sue Kenney's My Camino
    – Sue Kenney

PERSONAL FINANCES
*Don't Borrow $Money$ Until
    You Read This Book*
    – Paul E Counter

POETRY
Loveplay – Joe Fromstein
    and Linda Stitt
Two Voices / A Circle of Love
    – Serena Williamson
    Adams

**POLITICS AND
    HISTORY**
*Prophets of Violence / Prophets of
    Peace* – Dr. K. Sohail
Turning Points – Ray Argyle

SELF-HELP
Love, Sex and Marriage
    – Dr. K. Sohail/
    Bette Davis
*The Art of Living in Your Green
    Zone*
    – Dr. K. Sohail
*The Art of Loving in Your
    Green Zone*
    – Dr. K. Sohail
*The Art of Working in Your
    Green Zone*
    – Dr. K. Sohail/
    Bette Davis

TRUE CRIME - POLICE
10-45 Spells Death
    – Kathy McCormack
    Carter
Life on Homicide
    - Former Police Chief Bill
    McCormack
The Myth of The Chosen One
    – Dr. K. Sohail

RECOMMENDED READING
FROM OTHER PUBLISHERS

HISTORY
An Amicable Friendship (Canadiana) – Jan Th. J. Krijff

RELIGION
From Islam to Secular Humanism – Dr.K. Sohail

BIOGRAPHY
Gabriel's Dragon – Arch Priest Fr. Antony Gabriel

EPIC POETRY
Pro Deo – Prof Ronald Morton Smith